WILDERNESS
MEDICAL SOCIETY
PRACTICE GUIDELINES
FOR WILDERNESS EMERGENCY CARE

WILDERNESS
MEDICAL SOCIETY

PRACTICE GUIDELINES
FOR WILDERNESS EMERGENCY CARE

Second Edition

Edited by William W. Forgey, M. D.

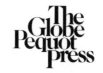

The
Globe
Pequot
Press

Guilford, Connecticut

Cover and text design: Lisa Reneson
Cover photo: Photodisc

Library of Congress Cataloging-in-Publication Data
Wilderness Medical Society practice guidelines for wilderness emergency care/edited by William W. Forgey.—2nd ed.
    p. cm.
  ISBN 0-7627-0671-6
  1. Mountaineering injuries. 2. First aid in illness and injury. 3. Wilderness survival. 4. Medical emergencies. I. Title: Practice guidelines for wilderness emergency care. II. Forgey, William W., 1942-

RC88.9.M6 W54 2000
616.02'5—dc21   00-055134

Manufactured in the United States of America
Second Edition/Third Printing

Table of contents

Appendices

Foreword

This is the fifth issue of the *Wilderness Medical Society Practice Guidelines for Wilderness Emergency Care*. The last issue was published in 1995, thus keeping to a five-year revision program. As seen in its predecessors, this issue contains both revised and new guidelines. This edition is the result of the identification of a need for clarification of prehospital care issues for injuries and illness that might be encountered in remote areas not serviced by normal response times of an emergency medical response system. The identification of topics was performed through the Society's continuing medical education process, from symposia sponsored by the Society, and from opinion obtained from identified experts.

New guidelines were drafted by James Schuler, D. O., and Stephanie Thompson, M. D., (Chapter 17: Botanical Encounters); Frank Butler, M. D., U.S.N. (Chapter 9: Wilderness Eye Injuries); and Ian Rogers, M.B.B.S., (Chapter 19: Marine Envenomations and Poisonings). Michael Cardwell and Ian Rogers made significant contributions to Chapter 20: Reptile Envenomation. David Johnson, M. D., made many recommendations and many others provided very pertinent updates to various existing guidelines. The Wilderness Eye Injury guideline enters new territory for the wilderness management of the eye. I believe that the Society is proposing an important advancement in remote area field care of ocular conditions.

Fifteen international experts identified in the Introduction reviewed these guidelines. Additional review and comments were sought for specific topics from additional Wilderness Society members. Those making significant contributions are also listed in the Introduction. The opinions contained in these guidelines do not represent the opinion of any state or governmental agency, even though some of the authors and reviewers are in government employ.

As with the last edition of the guidelines, the medical responses advocated herein do not delineate "levels of care," listing different appropriate responses for the lay public, paramedics, and advanced providers. The Society feels that there is an appropriate response to the various subjects selected, and that this response should be taught to anyone potentially responsible for backcountry medical care. This concept takes us the next logical step beyond standard urban first aid to a new first aid—a wilderness first aid. While various levels of wilderness medical care are being taught by many proprietary organizations, it is expected that when specific topics are selected that they include the advice provided by these guidelines.

William W. Forgey, M. D.
Editor, Practice Guidelines
President, Wilderness Medical Society
3595 East Fountain Boulevard, Suite A1
Colorado Springs, CO 80910

Introduction

"Wilderness," wrote E. O. Wilson, eminent Harvard professor, "settles peace on the soul because it needs no help; it is beyond human contrivance. Wilderness is a metaphor for unlimited opportunity."[1]

Many of us can identify with Wilson's expression of personal need and love for wilderness. We also know that in places that lie geographically far from definitive care, medical problems may arise that many of us are not trained to deal with appropriately. The purpose of the *Practice Guidelines* of the Wilderness Medical Society is to propose appropriate prehospital medical management for a variety of environmental and traumatic injuries that might be encountered during various wilderness activities. These practice guidelines do not reflect state laws concerning health care practices or licensure.

The guidelines are merely suggestions; your personal level of training, experience, and expertise will determine your willingness and ability to put into practice what is recommended in this book. If you travel into wilderness (defined as a remote geographical location more than one hour from definitive medical care) with the medical responsibility for a group, it is further recommended—on a moral, ethical, and legal basis—that you acquire the needed training, experience, and expertise before going.

The Wilderness Medical Society has made every effort to ensure the accuracy and appropriateness of these recommendations. It has utilized the expert opinion of specific individuals as well as workshops at each of the annual meetings since the last edition, for general membership input into the content of this edition. Members of the Society's Publications Committee and the Board of Directors performed a final review of content. It is anticipated that the review process will continue and that new guidelines will be issued in four years.

[1] Wilson, E.O. *The Diversity of Life.* Cambridge: Harvard University Press, 1992.

The Wilderness Medical Society wishes to thank members who contributed, some of them many long hours, to these position statements:

Wayne Askew, Ph.D.

Howard Backer, M.D.

Richard Banta, M.D.

Frank Butler, M.D., U.S.N.

Michael Cardwell

Lily Conrad, M.D.

Richard Dart, M.D.

Fred Darvill, Jr., M.D.

Steve Donelan

Blair Erb, M.D.

Edward Geehr, M.D.

Gordon Giesbrecht, Ph.D.

Paul Gill, Jr., M.D.

Philip Goodman, M.D.

Melissa Gray

Colin Grissom, M.D.

Peter Hackett, M.D.

Kenneth Iserson, M.D.

David E. Johnson, M.D.

Linda Lindsey, R.N.

Michael Mackan, M.D.

James Mohle, M.D.

Ian Rogers, M.B.B.S.

Ramon Ryan, M.D.

Tod Schimelpfenig

Joseph Serra, M.D.

James Shuler, D.O., M.S.

Jay Skidmore, Ph.D.

Daniel Spaite, M.D.

John Sullivan, M.D.

Stephanie Thompson, M.D.

Ken Zafren, M.D.

Review and approval of these guidelines was performed by members of the Publications Committee (Bruce Paton, M.D; R. Scott Hammond, M.D; Karl Neuman, M.D.; David Linn, M.D.; Matthew Russell, M.D.; David Townes, M.D., M.P.H.) and the Board of Directors (Robert Allen, M.D.*; Paul Auerbach, M.D.; Lily Conrad, M.D.; Anne Dickison, M.D.; Luanne Freer, M.D.*; Linda Lindsey, R.N.; Edward Otten, M.D.; Robert Schoene, M.D.; and Ken Zafren, M.D.*).

*Also denotes membership on the Publications Committee

Chapter 1

WILDERNESS EVACUATION

I. GENERAL INFORMATION

The mode and urgency of the evacuation should be appropriate for the problem. Calling for on-site evacuation, e.g., helicopter, versus evacuating a patient to care by foot or on a litter is decided in view of multiple factors including:

1) severity of the illness or injury
2) rescue and medical skills of the rescuers
3) physical/psychological condition of the rescuers and/or victim(s), including the motivation of the group to care for the patient and possibly alter trip plans, timetables, and goals
4) availability of equipment and/or aid for the rescue
5) the danger/difficulty of extracting the victim(s) by the various means available
6) time, a product of distance, terrain, weather, and multiple other variables
7) cost

An evacuation deemed necessarily "urgent" considers the patient's life or significant morbidity to be at immediate risk. A rescue is also deemed urgent if there is a similarly significant threat to rescuers. These guidelines indicate nonurgent evacuation in cases when the patient requires further evaluation and treatment but is not at immediate risk for significant morbidity or death.

Party leaders must know the capabilities of rescue organizations in the area the group is using and how to contact those organizations. All wilderness leaders must leave trip plans with a responsible person who can act in the group's behalf. If rescue by an outside group (rather than self-rescue by the party) has been determined to be the best course of action, the earlier it is initiated the better. Waiting may allow deterioration of the weather or the patient and may jeopardize the entire rescue operation.

When requesting outside assistance, the safety of incoming rescuers, their time commitment, and the cost of the rescue must be considered. It is important to note that the safety of the rescuers or the group takes precedence over ideal management of the patient. Optimally, the entire group, including the patient, must make evacuation decisions. The potential ecological damage that can occur to the wilderness rescue site from large numbers of rescuers entering the area would argue additionally in favor of self-rescue, if possible.

In general, it is appropriate to postpone further travel and/or initiate evacuation from the wilderness for any person who has the following:

1) Sustained or progressive physiological deterioration, manifested by orthostatic dizziness, syncope, tachycardia, bracycardia, dyspnea, altered mental status, progressive or significant weakness, intractable vomiting and/or diarrhea, inability to tolerate oral fluids, or the return of loss of consciousness following head injury. In other words, if patients are not improving, they must get out!

2) Debilitating pain

3) Inability to sustain travel at a reasonable pace due to a medical problem

4) Passage of blood by mouth or rectum, if not from an obviously minor source

5) Signs and symptoms of serious high altitude illness

6) Infections that progress for more than twenty-four hours despite the administration of appropriate treatment

7) Chest pain that is not clearly musculoskeletal in origin

8) The development of a psychological status that impairs the safety of the person or the group

Travel may continue if it is toward definitive care in the case of points 3, 4, and 8, or when descending in the case of point 5.

II. GUIDELINES FOR GROUND EVACUATION

If the decision has been made for a member of the party to walk out to obtain definitive care, the individual must not go alone unless there is no safe alternative. Whenever possible, at least two members of the party who are mentally and physically equipped to do so must accompany the patient.

If anything more complex than a simple walkout of the patient is required, e.g., a litter carry, an on-site leader must be identified who will assume responsibility for the evacuation. If an outside rescue is to be requested, a decision must be made on the most efficacious method of requesting this help. This will often require sending one, preferably two, members of the party to notify authorities that assistance is needed. This request must be carried in writing and include an assessment of the patient; overview of the situation including equipment, personnel, food, water; and a detailed location (map preferred) of the patient. The note should also include potential hazards to rescuers, limitations for vehicles, and so forth. Experience has shown that taking the time to write out a detailed note actually decreases total evacuation time. In assessing the anticipated length of evacuation time, the note must include the expertise and rescue experience of the persons in the field with the victim. In many countries a method of payment must be indicated before a rescue will be made.

During a litter evacuation, at least four and preferably six bearers must handle the litter at all times, except when doing so is physically impossible, such as carries over a narrow bridge. Additional personnel must be available to relieve those handling the litter. The number of litter carriers will ideally be eight persons per 100 meters (approximately 300 feet) of travel over rough terrain and six persons per 100 meters over reasonably smooth trail. It is very demanding to carry a loaded litter for more than fifteen to twenty minutes without rotating porters or taking a significant break. Litter carries, especially over rugged terrain, can be agonizingly slow. One bearer will be in charge of the litter, directing lifting and moving, directing the passing of the litter over obstacles, and assuming responsibility for continuously monitoring and reassuring the patient. Many teams standardize the position at the left front of the litter as the litter "driver's" position.

The patient must be carefully "packaged" in the litter for maximum safety and comfort. Protect the patient's head and eyes. Pad stress points, e.g., where the straps press against the body, and the voids, in the small of the back and behind the knees. Protect from wind, cold, and precipitation. To prevent decubitus ulcers, have the patient move occasionally or alter the patient's position at least every two hours if he or she is unconscious. Expect to handle urine and fecal elimination by allowing the functional patient to leave the stretcher with assistance (if serious spine injuries can be cleared), or provide appropriate tilting and/or cleansing toweling to catch excrement. To prevent deep vein thrombosis, allow leg movement or move or massage legs hourly, as long as this does not increase the severity of the original injury. If the litter is improvised, test the system and padding first on an uninjured person.

III. GUIDELINES FOR HELICOPTER EVACUATION

Helicopters can significantly reduce the time to definitive care when used for emergency transportation of the sick or injured. The decision to use a helicopter for an evacuation must take into account clinical, logistical, and environmental factors. Using a helicopter always adds an element of risk both to rescuers and victim, and a note requesting an air evacuation should include all known specific hazards relative to the rescue. This risk must be balanced against the risk to the patient, other members of the party, or the rescue team if the patient is evacuated by ground. Evacuate by helicopter only if: 1) a victim's life will be saved, 2) the victim has a significantly better chance for full recovery via a helicopter evacuation, 3) the pilot believes that conditions are safe enough to do the evacuation, 4) a ground evacuation may be unusually dangerous to the ground crew, 5) ground evacuation would be excessively prolonged, or 6) there are not enough rescuers available for a ground evacuation.

Four important points must be kept in mind: 1) evacuating a patient by ground may be faster than waiting for a helicopter (especially in high-risk flight conditions); 2) begin evacuation by ground if the helicopter may not be able to respond, or if removal from the accident site would benefit the patient, e.g., descent for altitude sickness; 3) patient may need to be moved to an appropriate landing site; and 4) do not use a helicopter to recover a corpse under emergency conditions.

A. Aircraft Limitations

Helicopters have various configurations, with different capabilities, and different crew skill levels. All helicopters are adversely affected by increased altitude, high environmental temperature, high wind, and heavy payload. The aircraft pilot makes the ultimate decisions concerning flight operations. A helicopter must not fly into known icing conditions or into even moderate storm conditions. Winds over forty-five mph, night flights into mountains, and landing in high winds are extremely hazardous. Not all helicopters or pilots are capable of flying by instruments into cloudy or foggy conditions. Party leaders must be familiar with ground-to-air signals, and if radio communication is available, the ground crew must keep the helicopter crew updated on weather and other related conditions at the scene.

Landing and taking off are the two most dangerous activities for both the air and ground crews. As altitude increases, the ability to make vertical hovers and land in small areas is greatly reduced. The optimal landing zone (LZ) is large, well marked, and relatively flat with a slope dropping slightly away from the LZ; has no tall objects on the perimeter; and has no loose debris that could be thrown up by the rapidly spinning blades. Marking at an LZ is best done with green reflective material; second best is red. The LZ may have to be prepared by the on-site personnel. It must be far enough from the patient so any maneuvering by the helicopter does not put the patient at risk. If there is no suitable landing zone, helicopters equipped for short haul or winch operations may be used.

The on-site personnel handling the patient must have some familiarity with helicopter operations. Helicopter landing zones are dangerous places. It is imperative to keep all nonessential personnel away from the area. If possible, assign personnel to keep a safe perimeter around the landing zone and to prevent people from approaching the craft. Wind generated by the helicopter is tremendous, and all ground personnel must protect themselves when the aircraft lands and takes off. In winter the wind chill from the rotor blades can cause frostbite. Never approach a helicopter until a signal has been given by one of the aircraft personnel. Never approach a helicopter from the rear where the spinning tail rotor is invisible and therefore dangerous, unless it is a rear-entry aircraft and the safe-approach signal has been clearly understood. Once on the ground, all directions from the aircraft crew must be followed explicitly.

B. Aeromedical Considerations

The mechanics and physiology of flight must be understood if it is to be safely used for patient transport. Noise and vibration levels are high, and it may be difficult to monitor or even communicate with the patient in flight without special equipment. Helicopter cabins are not pressurized. Atmospheric and oxygen pressure go down as the aircraft goes up. Supplemental oxygen must be available for all patients. Medical devices with air bladders, e.g., MAST, air splints, and endotracheal tubes, must be monitored for overinflation. Ground transport may be a safer alternative for patients with a suspected pneumothorax, decompression sickness, or air embolism.

IV. CONTROVERSIES

A. Is it appropriate to request aided evacuation from the wilderness? Evacuations from the wilderness create risk for the rescuers—who must walk or fly in—and are typically very expensive. It is improper to ask for help out of convenience when a group could carry out a self-rescue. In the United States, it is often assumed that a cry for help will bring an immediate response, free of charge. The "right" to free rescue is not guaranteed.

Especially in less developed countries, it is not always ethical to call for assistance since many native peoples require but cannot afford a lifesaving evacuation. Groups traveling into wilderness regions must be able to evacuate themselves. Request assistance as a last resort, when life or limb is threatened, or when the group is unable to carry out its own rescue.

B. Should helicopters be utilized in wilderness areas? Wilderness is a place where humans and their conveniences are a transient phenomenon, leaving little or no sign of their passing. Helicopters are an intrusion into wilderness, and the implications of nonessential use of helicopters in wilderness areas are an ethical issue.

Chapter 2

CARDIOPULMONARY RESUSCITATION

I. GENERAL INFORMATION

Guidelines for the general uses of cardiopulmonary resuscitation (CPR) are well defined, regularly updated, and widely distributed. Because the wilderness may impose circumstances that require special considerations in CPR, the following guidelines have been developed.

A. Contraindications to CPR in the Wilderness

There is no reason to initiate CPR if there is: 1) detection of vital signs; 2) danger to rescuers; 3) dependent lividity; 4) rigor mortis; 5) obvious lethal injury; 6) a well-defined Do Not Resuscitate (DNR) status; or 7) a patient with a rigid frozen chest. Criteria 3 and 4 may be difficult to evaluate in the nonfrozen, yet profoundly hypothermic person (see below) and without documentation criteria 6 is impossible to determine.

B. Discontinuation of CPR in the Wilderness

Once initiated, continue CPR until: 1) resuscitation is successful; 2) rescuers are exhausted; 3) rescuers are placed in danger; 4) patient is turned over to more definitive care; or 5) patient does not respond to prolonged (approximately thirty minutes) of resuscitative efforts (see Specific Situations, below).

C. Rescue Breathing

Initiate rescue breathing when a patient presents with ineffective breathing.

II. SPECIFIC SITUATIONS

A. Hypothermia

A cold, rigid, apparently pulseless and breathless patient is not necessarily a dead patient. If you fail to find respiration, initiate rescue breathing immediately. The patient needs oxygen, and there is **no** danger to the patient from rescue breathing. A cold patient with no detectable pulse should not necessarily be given chest compressions. Apparent pulselessness may be caused by hypothermia and the resulting tissue rigidity in combination with a very slow heart rate. Chest compressions may trigger ventricular fibrillation and will not be effective in someone dead from the cold. Do not initiate chest compressions in a patient with a rigid, frozen chest. Rescue breathing, preferably with supplemental oxygen, and immediate gentle evacuation are indicated. Do not use intermittent chest compressions as this technique may induce ventricular fibrillation, further compromising the circulation. If it is decided to initiate chest compressions, this technique must be continued by rescuers without interruption until the victim arrives at the Emergency Department.

B. Avalanche Victims

Breathless and pulseless victims of avalanches are usually dead from suffocation and/or blunt trauma. Hypothermia is often a confounding factor. Clear the airway, protect the cervical spine, and initiate rescue breathing and chest compressions (CPR) immediately.

Triage avalanche victims without vital signs at the scene according to the criteria of the International Commission for Alpine Rescue (ICAR) Medical Commission:

1) If there is no pulse and core temperature is 32°C (90°F) or above or burial is less than thirty minutes, continue CPR for twenty minutes. If successful with CPR, transfer to a hospital with an Intensive Care Unit. If unsuccessful, stop CPR.

2) If the core temperature is below 32°C (90°F) and burial is over thirty minutes, treatment depends upon the presence of an air pocket (any space around the nose or mouth, no matter how small):

   a) If an air pocket is present, continue CPR and transfer to a hospital with cardiopulmonary bypass capability

   b) If no air pocket is present, stop CPR

   c) If an air pocket is possible, but not certain, continue and transfer to a hospital with cardiopulmonary bypass capability or to a closer hospital where potassium can be measured. Patients with serum potassium greater than 10 mmol/L have no chance of survival and are declared dead by asphyxiation

C. Cold-Water Submersion

Near-drowning patients have occasionally been successfully resuscitated after prolonged (greater than thirty minutes) submersion in cold water (5 to 10°C or 41 to 50°F), but not without Advanced Life Support intervention. Successful resuscitation and favorable outcome are associated with young age, clean water, cold water, short duration of immersion, and pulse present or returning on scene with rescue breathing. Immediately initiate chest compressions and rescue breathing (CPR) and continue for at least thirty minutes.

D. Lightning Strike

Initiate rescue breathing and chest compressions (CPR) immediately on all pulseless, breathless victims of a lightning strike. Following a severe electrical shock, respiratory paralysis may persist long after cardiac activity returns. Rescuers must be prepared to provide prolonged resuscitation. If there are multiple victims, alter normal triage principles, i.e., treat seemingly dead victims first.

Chapter 3

SUBMERSION INJURIES

I. GENERAL INFORMATION

Rescue of a near-drowning victim is inherently dangerous. The following guidelines are suggested for getting the victim safely out of the water:

1) *Reach* for the victim, if possible, with an extended arm or leg, clothing, a stick or paddle, or anything that allows the rescuer to stay safely on land or in a boat.
2) When reaching is not possible, *throw* something that floats to the victim.
3) Throw a line to the victim and *tow* the victim to safety.
4) *Row* or paddle out to drowning victims, in a boat, wearing a personal flotation device.
5) Swimming rescues are extremely dangerous and are not recommended unless the rescuer has been trained and fully understands the risk involved. Do not attempt underwater searches for missing victims.

II. GUIDELINES FOR ASSESSMENT AND TREATMENT

Assess unconscious patients immediately for adequate respiration. This can sometimes be done in the water, if the rescuer is a strong swimmer and/or if the rescuer can stand in shallow water. Begin rescue breathing as soon as possible. There is no value in attempting to clear the patient's lungs of water but be prepared to roll the patient and clear the airway should water fill the airway during the rescue, or if the patient vomits.

Protect the spine of unconscious patients and of victims of diving or surfing accidents. In the absence of a pulse, begin chest compressions as soon as possible. Evaluate all drowning and near-drowning patients for hypothermia. Hypothermic submersion patients cannot be presumed dead until they are "warm and dead."

Urgently evacuate all submersion patients to definitive medical care. Even if the victim feels "ok," it is possible to develop delayed respiratory, renal, or other problems, so that evacuation is still indicated. Remember: Immediate treatment primarily by ventilation at the scene is the most important factor in determining survival.

III. CONTROVERSIES

A. Should all victims of accidental submersion be evacuated? Someone who is unexpectedly submersed and who comes up coughing but never loses consciousness does not need to be evacuated.

B. Should the Heimlich maneuver be used to clear the airway of a near-drowned victim? The American Heart Association unequivocally recommends an immediate start of CPR without the Heimlich maneuver in the case of a submersion victim. Utilize the Heimlich maneuver only if foreign matter is suspected of obstructing the airway or when attempts to ventilate the patient fail due to a blocked airway.

Chapter 4

HEAD INJURY

I. GENERAL INFORMATION

Anyone with a blow to the head or face, whether blunt or penetrating, risks developing increased intracranial pressure (ICP) or intracranial bleeding (ICB). Because definitive management of increasing ICP or ICB is not possible in the wilderness, prevention of head injuries should rank high among priorities. Prevention involves attention to safety and includes wearing an adequate helmet approved for the specific activity being undertaken. It must fit the user and be held in place with a nonstretching chinstrap. The use of even a properly fitted helmet does not preclude the possibility of a serious head injury, but it does reduce the risk. Chinstraps should not obstruct venous blood flow as this may cause ICP.

II. GUIDELINES FOR ASSESSMENT

Some individuals, after a blow to the head or face, are at low risk and do not need immediate evacuation. These patients have had a relatively trivial injury. They do not lose consciousness or lose consciousness for only a brief period of time. They have no history of a bleeding disorder or the use of medications that might increase the risk of bleeding. Monitor patients in this category for twenty-four hours and awaken every two hours for assessment. Watch for: 1) alterations in mental status, including personality changes, lethargy, drowsiness, disorientation, unusual irritability, and combativeness; 2) persistent nausea and vomiting; 3) change in visual acuity; and 4) alterations in coordination and/or speech. If these signs or symptoms of increasing ICP appear, then an evacuation should be initiated.

Immediate evacuation is recommended for all patients who have received a blow to the head or face that results in loss of consciousness for more than a brief period of time, who have significant signs or symptoms of increasing ICP, or have a depressed or basilar skull fracture. These signs and symptoms include:

1) debilitating headache
2) alterations in mental status (see above)
3) persistent nausea and vomiting
4) Battle's sign (ecchymosis behind and below the ears)
5) raccoon eyes (periorbital ecchymosis)
6) loss of coordination
7) loss of visual acuity
8) appearance of clear fluid (possibly cerebral spinal fluid) from the nose and/or ears
9) seizures
10) relapse into unconsciousness

III. GUIDELINES FOR TREATMENT

If there is an obvious head injury consider the possibility of a cervical spine injury (see Spinal Injury, Chapter 5). Specific measures to implement during evacuation include the critical importance of establishing and maintaining an airway in all unconscious patients. Airway management, without specific adjuncts, can usually be accomplished by keeping the patient in a stable side position, which also helps alleviate the possibility of aspirating vomitus, a common threat with head-injured patients. Alternatively, with consideration for possible spinal injury, place the patient with his/her head elevated approximately thirty degrees to decrease the chance of aspiration and to decrease ICP.

While all persons with a mechanism of injury that includes head trauma are strapped to a backboard in an urban setting, this is not necessary in the wilderness if the patient assessment does not indicate that evacuation is required. When evacuation is initiated, periodically reassess the requirement for neck or spine immobilization. If the spine can be cleared, terminate rigid immobilization even though the evacuation process is continued.

IV. CONTROVERSIES

A. Does any loss of consciousness following a blow to the head warrant evacuation of the patient? If the patient has been unconscious for only a brief period of time and/or with no obvious evidence of brain injury (see above), the patient may remain in the wilderness and be carefully monitored for twenty-four hours.

B. What is meant by "a brief period of time" in relation to unconsciousness? Seldom, if ever, is a period of unconsciousness accurately timed. The patient and/or witnesses are often unsure when unconsciousness occurred. Many authorities feel that a loss of consciousness for less than thirty seconds qualifies as a brief period of time, but consensus was not reached on this topic.

Chapter 5

SPINAL INJURY

I. GENERAL INFORMATION

In an urban environment, many patients placed in full spinal immobilization will prove to be free of unstable spine injuries. The inconvenience to patients and rescuers is worth the extra effort to protect the few patients with unstable spines. In wilderness situations, spinal immobilization is difficult and can drastically alter the logistics of an evacuation. Immobilize all patients with signs or symptoms as indicated in the Assessment and Treatment section below. Patients with no signs or symptoms need not be immobilized despite significant mechanisms of injury.

II. GUIDELINES FOR ASSESSMENT AND TREATMENT

In the wilderness a number of steps are involved in ruling out a spinal injury in a patient with a significant mechanism of injury. Treatment consists of full immobilization in a rigid litter, or immobilization with a cervical collar on the most level ground available until a rigid litter can be improvised or brought in.

Before deciding to clear the spine, finish a full secondary assessment to assure the patient has no obvious signs and symptoms of spine injury and to assess the patient for distracting injuries. Distracting injuries are any conditions that cause pain or which might affect the patient's mental alertness. Conditions such as significant blood loss, alcohol use, fractures, or disturbed psychological status are a few examples. It is recommended that the rescuer perform a second and specific assessment relative to the spine before making the decision to clear the spine. The cervical spine can be clinically cleared if **all** of the following are met and documented:

1) The patient must be fully awake and alert, with no alcohol or medications that might alter his or her level of consciousness.
2) The patient has no distracting injuries.

3) The patient has a completely normal motor and sensory neurological examination.

4) There is no pain or tenderness to palpation of the posterior cervical area and no palpable step-off deformity.

5) There is no pain on unassisted range of motion of the neck.

III. CONTROVERSIES

Should all patients with a suspected spinal injury be immobilized and evacuated? In the wilderness, full spinal immobilization may pose unnecessary hardship and danger to patients and rescuers. Therefore, seek a balance between the difficulties and dangers of evacuating an immobilized patient on one hand and not immobilizing a spinal injury on the other. In certain hazardous situations, it may be safer for the patient and rescuers to forego spinal immobilization, or to use only partial spinal immobilization such as a cervical collar alone, to evacuate more easily and rapidly from the area of immediate danger.

Chapter 6

WILDERNESS WOUND MANAGEMENT

I. GENERAL INFORMATION

Assume contamination of open wounds and treat accordingly. The major goals are: 1) stop blood loss; 2) clean the wound and keep it clean; 3) promote healing and reduce discomfort; and 4) minimize loss of function. Most wilderness first aid kits contain simple bandages and compresses only. Improvisation and the use of substitute materials are often required. Wilderness wounds are at risk for tetanus. Ensuring current tetanus immunization prior to participation in wilderness activities is encouraged.

II. GUIDELINES FOR ASSESSMENT AND TREATMENT

Wear fluid barrier gloves when contacting blood or other body fluids, unless a delay to obtain them would be harmful to the patient. Improvised personal protection could include, for example, a plastic food bag or piece of garment to minimize contact with the victim's blood and sunglasses or ski goggles to protect your eyes.

Even heavy bleeding can be controlled with pressure techniques in nearly all instances. Initially, apply direct digital pressure over the bleeding vessels and elevate the wound. Alternately, stop severe bleeding by placing two fingers, held together, into the wound. This temporary stasis is continued through the use of an internal pressure dressing made by taking a moist wad of gauze or clean cloth and packing it firmly into the wound. This is held in position with strips of gauze or tape. These strips are not circumferentially tight but just cover and hold the packing gauze in place. Pressure points alone are not effective as a primary technique to control bleeding but may be useful as an adjunct. Arterial tourniquets are rarely necessary and, if used, must be released approximately every five minutes, while continuing to apply direct wound pressure, to assess the continued need for the tourniquet.

A. Contusions

During the first forty-eight hours, contusions may be treated with cold compresses or cold-water immersion and a compression dressing, to limit expanding hematomas and to aid in pain relief. Apply cold for one-half hour every two hours with due regard to possible cold injury. After seventy-two hours, apply heat in the same manner to promote healing. Topical heat ointments or creams can cause skin irritation; their use is discouraged. Large contused areas with marked swelling cause severe pain and disability and may signal a large amount of blood loss or a significant underlying injury. Evaluate such patients for shock and other possible injuries and treat accordingly. Do not drain hematomas. A major soft tissue injury in proximity to a bone should arouse a high suspicion of a fracture. Apply splints for comfort.

B. Subungual Hematomas

May be drained by drilling a hole in the nail with a red-hot paper clip, a sharp blade, or hypodermic needle to provide pain relief.

C. Abrasions

May be cleaned with soap and water or with a surgical scrub such as .5% chlorhexidine gluconate or a 1% povidone-iodine impregnated sponge, both diluted with water. Follow scrubbing with copious irrigation with clean water. Water safe to drink is clean enough for wound cleaning. After the abrasion has been cleaned, apply a thin coating of a topical antimicrobial first-aid ointment and dress with sterile gauze. If water is in short supply, the simple application of antibiotic ointment within three hours significantly reduces wound infection.

D. Lacerations and Avulsions

Use copious irrigation with clean water. Use water that is potable, unless the wound is grossly contaminated and no other irrigation is available. Boiled then cooled water is safest for open fractures or joints. Pressure irrigation with a syringe and needle or a barrel irrigation syringe is the most effective technique. Improvised equipment could include a plastic bag with a hole the size of a pencil in it. Irrigate with at least 500 ml of water. Take care to avoid splashing fluid into the irrigator's face. Following irrigation, inspect the wound and remove remaining debris with a sterile (flamed or boiled) forceps.

Do not close heavily contaminated or high-risk wounds because of the increased chance of wound infection. Pack heavily contaminated wounds open with wet-to-dry dressings. Wounds that open into joint spaces, that involve underlying tendons and ligaments, that open the face (for cosmetic reasons), that affect areas of special function (e.g., hands), and bites from wild animals (see Wild Land Animal Attacks, Chapter 18) are best cleaned and dressed without closure and the patient evacuated for definitive care. If evacuation is not feasible, or will take longer than two days, it is reasonable to treat significant wounds with thorough cleaning and closure with tape, wound closure strips, sutures, or surgical staples. Minor wounds do not require urgent evacuation and may be closed with tape or wound closure strips. Limit sharp debridement to obviously devitalized tissue. Splinting and elevation will help maintain wound closure, hemostasis, and pain control, although this is probably only feasible under limited circumstances.

If bone is exposed or if the wound is a deep puncture or highly contaminated, give appropriate antibiotics.

Traumatic amputations necessitate proper management of the amputated part, if there will be any opportunity for re-implantation. Gently clean the amputated part and wrap in slightly moist sterile gauze, seal in plastic, and keep as cool as possible without freezing (ice water is best). Some parts, such as fingers, may be reattached up to thirty-two hours after the injury.

Ascertain tetanus status and give recommendations for updating after leaving the wilderness. Observe wounds daily for signs of infection, that indicate the need for further irrigation drainage, or debridement.

E. Impaled Objects

Remove impaled objects at the scene. Strong resistance or severely increasing pain on attempts at removal are a contraindication to removal. Stabilizing in place is virtually impossible. The risk of continued bleeding and continued damage to underlying structures outweighs the possibility of damage resulting from removal.

III. GUIDELINES FOR EVACUATION

Rapid evacuation from the wilderness is advisable for:

1) severe animal bites or bites from potentially rabid animals
2) deep or highly contaminated wounds with a high risk of infection
3) wounds that open to fractures (other than the distal phalanx) or to joint spaces

4) infected wounds not responding to reasonable field treatment

5) wounds associated with severe blood loss

While not an urgent matter, consider evacuation for wounds that severely limit an individual's ability to participate in the trip and wounds that require closure for cosmetic reasons (such as wounds on the face). Delayed primary closure of facial wounds can be performed in three to five days if the wound is kept clean with daily packing.

IV. CONTROVERSIES

A. Should wounds be closed in the wilderness? Although sterile techniques are virtually impossible in the wilderness, primary closure with sutures, staples, surgical/wound glue or wound closure strips may be feasible for relatively clean wounds. Staples provide a cosmetic result identical to that of interrupted sutures, but not subcuticular sutures. The patient's comfort and ability and willingness to function are increased, and healing time is usually shortened. For ulcerations, abscess cavities, deep puncture wounds, and animal bites, do not close wounds but allow to gradually heal by granulation and eventual re-epithelization. Wounds grossly contaminated with soil or feces must be cleaned and observed for four to five days before closure if the wilderness trip lasts that long.

B. Should antibiotic prophylaxis be considered for wilderness wounds? The following are general indications for antibiotic prophylaxis:

1) significantly contaminated wounds requiring extensive cleaning and debridement (especially in patients with pre-existing valvular heart disease, prosthetic joints, or immunosuppressed patients);

2) violation of cartilage, joint spaces, tendon, or bone;

3) crush-mechanism wounds with a high potential for devitalization;

4) mammalian bites (see Wild Land Animal Attacks, Chapter 18).

For prophylaxis use amoxicillin clavulanate, a second or third generation cephalosporin, a quinolone, a penicillinase resistant penicillin, or a tetracycline antibiotic. Five days of prophylactic therapy suffice.

Chapter 7

BURN MANAGEMENT

I. GENERAL INFORMATION

The most likely source of major burn trauma in the outdoors is from flammable fuel used in camp stoves and lanterns. Scalds from hot liquids can also cause extensive burns. Thermal injuries from stoves, carbide lights and lanterns, hot utensils, and campfires are generally not extensive. Stress the importance of prevention.

II. GUIDELINES FOR ASSESSMENT AND TREATMENT

Every aspect of burn treatment depends on assessment of the depth and extent of the injury. Although this assessment may be an estimate, it is the basis for deciding how the patient will be treated, whether evacuation is required, and, if so, how urgently.

A. Assessment

Depth: Superficial burns involve the epidermis only. The skin color is red to pale and no blister forms. Partial thickness burns have blisters in addition to the red discoloration of the skin. Full thickness burns have a pale or charred skin color and do not have blister formation.

Extent: Use the Rule of Nines, in which each arm represents approximately 9 percent of a person's total body surface area (TBSA), each leg 18 percent (the front of the leg 9 percent, and the back of the leg 9 percent), the front of the torso represents 18 percent, the back of the trunk 18 percent, the head represents 9 percent, and the groin 1 percent. For infants and small children, the head represents a larger percentage (18 percent) and the legs a smaller percentage (13.5 percent). For smaller areas, use the Rule of Palmar Surface: the patient's entire palmar surface (surface of palm and fingers) equals about 1 percent TBSA.

Pain: In addition to depth and extent, also include an assessment of pain. Adequate control of pain is a treatment goal and indicator of the ability to manage a burn wound while in the wilderness. If you cannot manage the pain, your treatment is inadequate.

B. Initial Care

1) Stop the burning process. The faster the better, within thirty seconds if possible. Heat can continue to injure tissue as long a material with a temperature above 65°C (149° F) is in contact with the skin. No first aid will be effective until the burning process has stopped. Smother flames, if appropriate, then cool the burn with water with due regard to causing hypothermia in an extensively burned patient. Remove clothing and jewelry from the burn area. Do not try to remove anything that has stuck to the wound.

2) Manage the ABCs.

3) Assess for associated injuries such as fractures or lacerations and inhalation injury.

4) Evaluate the burn (depth, extent, and pain).

5) General treatment for the patient:

    a) Stabilize the body temperature. When skin is lost, so is the patient's ability to thermoregulate.

    b) Elevate injured parts.

    c) Hydration is of critical importance in long-term care. Have the patient drink as much fluid as he/she can tolerate, unless the patient complains of nausea. Avoid vomiting, if possible. Include some salt in the oral fluids, but do not make these solutions stronger than .9%.

    d) Remember: Altered consciousness is due to a cause other than the burn.

C. General Treatment of the Burn

Caring for the wound itself is often the least important aspect of burn care. All burn wounds are sterile for the first twenty-four to forty-eight hours. Burn management is aimed primarily at keeping the wound clean and reducing the pain.

1) Gently wash the burn with slightly warm water and mild soap, if needed, to remove any debris and to clean the skin surface around the burn site. Pat dry. Remove the skin from blisters that have popped open or are hemorrhagic (but do not open blisters).

2) Dress burns with a thin layer of antibiotic ointment.

3) Cover the burn with Spenco 2nd Skin or a similar dressing if the burn is small enough, or cover with a thin layer of gauze, or with clean, dry clothing. The use of hyperosmolar solutions such as honey or sugar is usable as a field expedient dressing. It has been suggested that honey would serve as a burn dressing. Covering wounds reduces pain and evaporative losses, but do not use an occlusive dressing.

4) When evacuation is imminent, do not redress or reexamine the injury. If evacuation is prolonged, redress once daily. Remove old dressings, reclean (removing the old ointment), and apply fresh ointment and a clean dry covering. (Note: soak off old dressings with clean, tepid water.)

5) Do not pack wounds in ice but cool with wet cloth bandages. Do not leave wet coverings on large burns for more than two hours at a time to reduce the risk of hypothermia.

6) Elevate burned extremities to minimize swelling. Swelling retards healing and encourages infection. Have the patient gently and regularly move burned areas as much as possible.

7) Ibuprofen is probably the best over-the-counter analgesic for burn pain (including sunburn).

8) If you have no ointment or dressings, leave the burn alone. The burn's surface will dry into a scab-like covering that provides protection.

III. GUIDELINES FOR EVACUATION

Superficial burns, even extensive ones, rarely require evacuation. Although they do not require rapid evacuation, blistered burns greater than 1 percent TBSA are difficult to keep clean in the wilderness and should be evacuated. Partial thickness burns covering less than 15 percent TBSA must receive definitive care but seldom warrant urgent evacuation. Full thickness burns need definitive medical care to heal best but do not usually require urgent evacuation unless they are extensive. Partial thickness and full thickness burns covering more than 15 percent TBSA are often a threat to life, requiring urgent evacuation. Any serious burn to the face may have burned the patient's airway and must be considered an urgent evacuation. Urgently evacuate patients with any burns to hands, feet or genitals. Urgently evacuate electrical or chemical burns.

Chapter 8

ORTHOPEDIC INJURIES

I. GENERAL INFORMATION

Sprains, strains, and fractures, especially injuries to lower extremities, are among the most common accidents in wilderness settings. The treatment of these injuries may vary, depending upon the expertise and experience of those in the party and the distance from definitive medical help. In remote settings, making the patient as functional as possible is often the overriding concern, thereby facilitating self-rescue and eliminating the need for outside assistance. Remember, the safety of the group takes precedence over optimal treatment of any individual injury.

Managing fractures in remote environments requires common sense, good diagnostic skills, and sensitivity to the needs of the patient and the group. For example, in a severe ankle injury where a fracture is suspected, one would normally immobilize the part and put the patient on crutches with instructions for elevation, ice, and rest from weight bearing. In the wilderness, however, one must weigh other factors: the desire of the patient to ambulate on a suspicious ankle injury, the availability of people to transport the patient, the type of terrain involved in transport, the severity of the environment, distance involved, and the patient's need or desire as well as ability to continue carrying a load. Thus, whereas the best medical judgment precludes weight bearing, the best decision in a remote environment might be to immobilize the ankle in a splint, or tape the ankle securely as for an athletic event, and allow the patient to hobble along on his or her good ankle using an ice axe, ski pole or wooden stick for balance. This could be the safest and most reasonable decision based on the situation.

II. GUIDELINES FOR ASSESSMENT AND TREATMENT: FRACTURES

In the wilderness, without a radiographic picture of the involved bones, assessment of a fracture includes the following questions:

1) Are there obvious signs of a fracture, such as angulations, swelling, or bruising?
2) Can the patient move the injury or does she/he guard it carefully?
3) Is there crepitation with movement?
4) Is there point tenderness with palpation of the site, or pain at the suspected injury site with axial compression along the long bone or with torque on the bone?
5) Is there discoloration and swelling?
6) How does the injured side compare to the uninjured side?
7) Does the injury feel rigid with spasm of the surrounding muscles?
8) Did the patient feel or hear anything break?
9) What was the mechanism of injury? (High-speed impacts cause more fractures than low-speed impacts).
10) Is there adequate circulation distal to the suspected fracture site?
11) How willing is the patient to use the injured area?

The key elements of a splint are adequate padding for comfort and adequate rigidity for safety. Splinting may be accomplished with formal splints or improvised splints, e.g., clothing, adhesive or athletic tape, foamlite sleeping pads, ice axes, ski poles, or natural material. The patient is the best source of information on how well splints are working. Peripheral pulses must be monitored before and after all splinting. Check pulses and distal limb color periodically to ensure that the splint wrap is not too tight. It is important to give the patient the responsibility of notifying someone of any changes in sensation or level of pain.

A. Shoulder

Fractures of the shoulder girdle are quite often stable and require nothing more than sling immobilization, cold compresses, if available, and allowance for gentle motion of the forearm and hand. A fracture of the clavicle may be treated with a sling and swathe. The hand and wrist must be accessible for feeling pulses.

B. Upper Arm

The humeral shaft is palpable on the medial side throughout its entire length. Therefore, when a fracture is suspected, palpate the length of the humerus, beginning either proximal or distal to the patient's area of complaint. In this way, very small, nondisplaced fractures may be identified.

Ask the patient to extend her or his wrist, digits, and thumb to check the radial nerve function and document for future reference. Immobilizing the arm against the body wall is nature's best splint. Humeral fractures can be very adequately padded and immobilized in this manner with a sling and swathe. For comfort leave the elbow free and dependent, allowing gravity to apply gentle traction to the fracture site, which is splinted to the thorax with only the swathe. An unstable or displaced humeral fracture may require a padded splint.

C. Lower Arm

Adequately splint fractures of the elbow, forearm, and wrist, incorporating the joints above and below. If possible, splint the elbow at eighty to ninety degrees of flexion to elevate the forearm and hand and reduce swelling.

The stability provided by a rigid splint is worth the effort, especially in a long and difficult transport. Splint fractures of the distal ulna and radius with the hand placed in the position of function with a rolled up sock, glove, or other soft material tucked into the palm. Then immobilize the hand, wrist, and forearm in a splint. Active exercise of the hand is quite helpful in promoting circulation.

Correct marked angulation. Applying a splint to a badly angulated forearm fracture is difficult and usually unstable. Gentle traction with an assistant applying counter-traction to the upper arm results in an overall improvement with a negligible risk of creating further vascular or neurologic damage. Move slowly and stop if force is required for further movement, or the patient complains of significantly increasing pain.

D. Hand

Fractures of the hand are often associated with dislocations of the proximal or distal interphalangeal joints. Reduce phalangeal fractures and splint in a position of function as indicated above, not in an extended position. Immediately after injury, these fractures can be reduced with only minimal discomfort. Hours after the injury, swelling and pain make realignment more difficult. Use of an ice compress and very gentle traction can realign fractures of the hand without significant discomfort. Immobilize the digits in a position of function whenever possible, and use adjacent digits for splinting (the "buddy system"). Place gauze between the buddy-taped fingers to absorb moisture. A suitable hand splint may be made by placing the hand in a functional position with a soft roll of material in the palm, and then wrapping the whole hand with an elastic wrap or roller gauze. Torn strips of clothing can be used for an improvised hand splint.

E. Hip

In fractures of the hip, the typical position of external rotation and short-ening of the leg may or may not be present. The fracture may be an impact-ed femoral neck type or an acetabular fracture. Diagnosis might be diffi-cult. As a general guideline, if a patient has sustained significant trauma and has very painful motion in the region of the hip, plus pain with weight bearing, carry him or her out on a litter or sled. Do not place suspected fractures of the hip in traction. Secure the leg on the affected side to the uninjured leg for splinting.

F. Pelvis

In suspected fractures of the pelvis, treat for shock due to the massive blood loss often associated with this injury. Because of possible bladder trauma, check for hematuria. Gentle constricting wraps placed around the pelvic region may provide temporary comfort and more stability to the fracture. A ThermaRest pad, secured around the pelvis then inflated, offers excellent improvised pelvic stability. The patient requires stabiliza-tion on a rigid backboard, litter, or sled.

G. Femur

Fractures of the femoral shaft must be treated in traction for many impor-tant reasons. The most important is that traction reestablishes normal length and conformity of the musculature and tightens the fascial enve-lope, which decreases the bleeding that occurs in the thigh. A patient with a femoral shaft fracture can easily lose more than a liter (two pints) of blood into the thigh and, if the fracture is movable and the thigh unsta-ble, this bleeding can continue. Additionally, fracture fragments may cause further vascular damage.

Traction also relieves pain, stabilizes fracture fragments, prevents converting a closed fracture into an open fracture, and reduces further soft-tissue damage. In a major expedition or an extended trek into remote regions, the expedition physician or paramedical person in charge must plan ahead for the type of traction that will be used if a femoral shaft frac-ture occurs. Commercial traction devices are lightweight, easy to use, and efficient.

Improvised femoral traction can be satisfactory, but must be prac-ticed prior to the actual event, or at least tried out on an uninjured volun-teer first, so that everyone understands and is familiar with the plan. Once a fractured femur has been diagnosed, assign someone to apply manual traction to the extremity (with the patient protected from the environment) until the traction device is in place. A general rule for how much traction to apply is 10 percent of the patient's body weight or until the pain is relieved. Additional immobilization of the fractured extremity to the uninjured leg with adequate padding can also be helpful. When long transport is anticipated, place padding behind the knee to create 5 to 10 percent knee flexion. This position is much more comfortable than if the knee is fully extended in traction.

Frequently monitor and document circulation distal to the injury. It is not necessary to remove the boot and sock in most instances and may be inadvisable in cold weather. Traction is usually more comfortable with the boot and sock on, and the dorsalis pedis pulse can usually be palpated by sliding a finger under the sock. A gross determination of sensation and skin warmth can be made by palpation. The patient can relate sensations of numbness or tingling in the toes. A complication of the traction splinting techniques that employ an ankle hitch is skin tissue necrosis of the ankle or foot. This can be avoided by padding beneath the ankle hitch, removing the traction splint for periods of time, or using tape-to-skin traction with the boot off instead of an ankle hitch.

H. Knee

Patellar fractures from a fall directly on the knee may be difficult to differentiate from a severe contusion unless there is an obvious deformity. A person with a compound fracture of the patella will be unable to extend the knee. Immobilize a patient with severe knee pain in a cylinder splint that stabilizes the knee and allows walking with assistance. Improvise a cane or crutch if terrain and other factors dictate that this is the best course of action.

I. Lower Leg

Splint tibia and both bone fractures to incorporate the knee and ankle. Many isolated fibula fractures require only an ankle splint and the victim can ambulate with a cane or crutch. Traction splinting is unnecessary. Gently correct angular deformities (see Lower Arm above).

J. Ankle

Fractures of the ankle may be difficult to assess. Early examination and treatment are important. Immobilize adequately, then elevate and apply cold to the injured extremity. A well-wrapped compression dressing is also quite helpful. Ankle fractures may be splinted very well with parkas, foam sleeping pads, or other comparable gear arranged in a U shape around the foot and lower leg.

III. GUIDELINES FOR ASSESSMENT AND TREATMENT: DISLOCATIONS

It is important to diagnose and reduce a dislocation quickly after it occurs. Discretion must obviously be used in deciding to reduce the dislocation when evacuation to a nearby medical facility can be easily accomplished.

The major advantages of early reduction are:

1) Reduction is easier immediately after the injury, before swelling and muscle spasm have developed
2) Transport of the patient is easier after reduction
3) Reduction usually results in dramatic pain relief
4) Immobilization of the injured joint is easier to accomplish and more stable after reduction
5) The safety of the entire party may be jeopardized during the evacuation of a patient with a major joint dislocation
6) Early reduction reduces the circulatory and neurological risks to the extremity

Signs helpful in identifying a dislocation include:

1) Restriction of motion through the joint's normal range
2) Obvious deformity in comparison with the uninvolved side
3) Crepitus or grating of bone fragments is absent
4) Often a typical, identifiable posture of the dislocated joint, which the patient will maintain to minimize pain

Obtaining a history of the mechanism of injury is helpful. Avulsion fractures may accompany dislocations. The alignment of these fractures is usually improved with the reduction of the dislocation. The same is true of vessel or nerve impairment associated with a dislocation. When a major long bone fracture (e.g., femur or humerus) accompanies a dislocation in the same area, the dislocation may not even be diagnosed in view of the more apparent major fracture. In these cases, splinting of the fracture is the main concern. The dislocation, for all practical purposes, is a secondary issue and usually not amenable to reduction by ordinary means.

A. Shoulder

Anterior-inferior dislocations of the shoulder joint account for over 90 percent of shoulder dislocations. The mechanism of injury is usually external rotation and abduction. The problem is often recurrent and the patient can identify the dislocation quite readily. The patient will usually stabilize the shoulder in the most comfortable position but cannot bring the involved extremity across the chest to a position of rest. The upper arm is held away from the body in various positions and cannot be brought into a sling-type position. This differentiates a dislocation from a fracture of the humerus, in which the patient usually splints the upper arm against the chest wall for comfort. Check circulation, motor and sensory function to the hand, and also sensory function along the outer aspect of the shoulder (axillary nerve), and document findings.

Posterior dislocations of the shoulder are not common. In this instance, the upper arm and forearm are held across the anterior chest wall and attempts at externally rotating the upper arm away from the chest are restricted and painful. The diagnosis is often difficult to make.

One method for reduction of an anterior shoulder dislocation is steady traction with the arm abducted ninety degrees, pulling straight from the body with counter-traction provided in the region of the axilla by an assistant. Muscle relaxation through massage can enhance attempts at relocation and is appropriate. Be sure to pad the axilla and the antecubital region to protect nerve and vascular structures during traction.

A second method is to place the patient prone and let the arm hang down toward the ground with ten to fifteen pounds of weight secured to the hand. This method may be slow and relaxation is critically important, but the muscles will generally fatigue in time, and manual assistance by manipulation of the shoulder is helpful.

After reduction, immobilize the shoulder with sling and swathe.

B. Elbow

Look for obvious deformity when compared to the uninvolved side and restricted flexion and extension of the joint. Most commonly, the olecranon dislocates toward the rear, and a bony prominence shows posteriorly.

Apply slow, steady traction to the forearm in a partially flexed position with counter-traction applied to the upper arm by an assistant. The patient's ability to fully flex the elbow is a sign of reduction. The joint may be displaced medially or laterally and may require side pressure for realignment. After reduction, immobilize in a sling and swathe. If reduction is not possible, splint in the position found.

C. Wrist

Wrist dislocations are very difficult to differentiate from a fracture, and often difficult to reduce. Splint immobilization is the treatment of choice (see Lower Arm, page 26). Circulation and neurologic function to the hand are usually not compromised; if they are, attempt reduction with gentle in-line traction.

D. Fingers

Obvious deformity and limited function are the main diagnostic factors. Reduction of dislocations of middle and distal interphalangeal joints is accomplished by maintaining the digit in partial flexion and pushing the dislocated base of the phalanx back in place while traction is applied to the partially flexed digit.

There are two hand dislocations in which reduction is difficult, if not impossible, by closed means: dislocation of the metacarpophalangeal joint of the index finger and the metacarpophalangeal joint of the thumb. The thumb is sometimes reducible closed, but the index metacarpal rarely is. Make one attempt, then immobilize the joint in a functional position. Do not persist with multiple attempts.

E. Hip

The majority of dislocations are posterior. The hip will be moderately flexed, internally rotated and adducted. Any attempt to extend the hip for splinting or easier transport will be resisted by the patient and is mechanically nearly impossible to accomplish. Anterior dislocation of the hip results in a posture of extension, external rotation and abduction. Again, attempting to extend the hip to a neutral position is very difficult, if not impossible, and is resisted by the patient.

If skill and equipment are available, the use of intramuscular or intravenous muscle relaxants or analgesics greatly facilitate any reduction. This reduction requires two people, ideally, with one applying counter-traction to the pelvis with the patient lying in a supine position on the ground. In the case of a posterior hip dislocation, the involved hip and knee are flexed to ninety degrees with the rescuer straddling the patient and applying traction in an upward direction. If only one person is available to attempt the reduction, the victim can be placed prone over a log, rock, or bench, and the traction applied downward with hip and knee flexed ninety degrees. Once reduced, the injured hip must be immobilized to the uninvolved extremity and the patient transported in a supine position.

F. Patella

Most often, the patella is laterally displaced with the knee held in flexion for comfort. Such an injury is often recurrent and caused by a pivoting type of injury with a partially flexed knee. The patella is not movable and is obviously out of place.

Flex the hip to relax the quadriceps, then apply gentle traction to extend the knee. In most cases, the patella will slip back into its groove.

Applying direct, gentle pressure to the patella from the lateral aspect may be necessary to attain reduction. Immobilize the extremity with a cylinder splint. With the knee extended and immobilized, the patient may be able to walk well enough for self-evacuation.

G. Knee

Major ligamentous disruption is the rule in dislocations of the knee. The knee may not be dislocated at the time of exam, but gross instability is the major clue, and vascular impairment is an important risk. Check pulses and motor function in ankle and foot.

Gentle realignment of the joint benefits damaged neurovascular structures. Splint securely, without compromising circulation to the foot. The patient must be carried out.

H. Ankle

Most commonly associated with fractures, the dislocated ankle is obviously deformed and often manifests crepitus. Reduce the deformity as much as possible as necrosis of tight, stretched overlying skin is a danger. Ordinarily, this is not difficult because of the gross instability resulting from associated fractures. Hold the forefoot and allow the remainder of the extremity to act as the counter-traction. Improved alignment of the ankle dislocation results without much additional effort. Gentle traction of the heel and foot also helps. Immobilize with a splint, and carry the patient out.

IV. GUIDELINES FOR EVACUATION

Deciding which injuries mandate premature termination of a trip, and how rapidly and by what means evacuation will be performed is a function of both the type of trip and type of injury. Urgent evacuation is indicated in: 1) open fractures; 2) injuries with vascular compromise not alleviated by reduction; 3) spinal injuries with neurologic deficits; and 4) injuries associated with significant blood loss. Evacuation is **not** needed for: digit injuries and minimal injuries to other joints. With adequate splinting, delays in reaching definitive medical care often result in no permanent harm.

Chapter 9

WILDERNESS EYE INJURIES

I. GENERAL INFORMATION

Management of ocular emergencies in the wilderness is made more difficult by three factors: 1) the lack of diagnostic equipment such as a slit lamp; 2) the lack of specialty consultation; and 3) limited medications with which to treat the disorders encountered. Typical of many wilderness medical management issues, the diagnostic and therapeutic approaches presented below are not necessarily to be used when professional referral is readily available.

This guideline discusses sudden vision loss in a noninflamed eye, orbital and periorbital inflammation, and acute red eye. The available medications and equipment with which to treat these disorders will be assumed to be those in the recommended wilderness ocular emergency kit shown below.

II. MEDICATIONS AND EQUIPMENT

The proposed management of ocular emergencies in the wilderness will require that the medications and equipment shown below are available to the treating medical personnel:

Wilderness Eye Kit Medications

Ciprofloxacin 0.3% drops
Tetracaine 0.5% drops
Prednisolone acetate 1% drops
Levofloxacin 500 mg tabs
Bacitracin ophthalmic ointment
Prednisone 20 mg tabs
Artificial tears
Scopolamine 0.25% drops
Diclofenac 0.1% drops
Pilocarpine 2% drops

Wilderness Eye Kit Equipment

Penlight with cobalt blue filter
Fluorescein strips
Cotton-tipped applicators
Metal eye shield (or rig from suitable material)
Eye patches (or equal)
1-inch tape
Wound closure strips (¼ inch) (or make from wider tape)
Magnifying glass

III. GUIDELINES FOR ASSESSMENT AND TREATMENT

When confronted by ocular disorders in the wilderness, attempt to measure the visual acuity. Reading the print in a book or any other printed material will provide at least a rough measure of visual acuity.

A. Acute Vision Loss in the Noninflamed Eye

Disorders that may cause acute visual loss in a noninflamed eye include retinal detachment, central retinal artery occlusion, anterior ischemic optic neuropathy, optic neuritis, central retinal vein occlusion, arteritic anterior ischemic optic neuropathy, vitreous hemorrhage, and significant high-altitude retinal hemorrhage. These disorders are difficult to diagnose and treat in the wilderness. In most cases, all that can be done is to arrange for an urgent evacuation.

Giant Cell Arteritis: A key question that must be asked is, "Does he or she have Giant Cell Arteritis (GCA)?" This is important because visual loss in one eye due to GCA is often rapidly followed by visual loss in the other eye if untreated. In addition, untreated GCA has a significant mortality. Diagnostic factors that may help to identify a person with GCA are age greater than fifty-five, temporal headache, jaw claudication, fever, weight loss, previous transient episodes of visual loss, and generalized muscle aches and fatigue. If GCA is suspected, start the individual on prednisone 80 mg a day and evacuate on an urgent basis.

Central retinal artery occlusion: The other cause of acute visual loss in a noninflamed eye that may sometimes be treated successfully in the wilderness is central retinal artery occlusion. For this reason, treat acute loss of vision in the wilderness with a trial of supplemental oxygen, if available, at the highest inspired fraction achievable as soon as possible after the onset of symptoms. If supplemental oxygen is to be of any benefit, a response is typically seen within just a few minutes.

B. Orbital or Periorbital Inflammation

This may result from preseptal cellulitis, orbital cellulitis, pseudotumor, insect envenomation, or dacryocystitis. Preseptal cellulitis is characterized by periocular erythema and edema, a history of periocular trauma or hordeolum, no proptosis, no restriction of extraocular motility, and no change in visual acuity. Treatment for preseptal cellulitis is levofloxacin 500 mg once a day with expedited evacuation if no improvement is seen in twenty-four to forty-eight hours.

Dacryocystitis is a specific type of preseptal cellulitis in which the source of the infection is an obstructed nasolacrimal duct. The erythema and inflammation are localized to the area overlying the lacrimal sac at the inferior nasal aspect of the lower eyelid. It is treated in the same manner as described above except that warm compresses should also be used. The diagnosis of periocular insect envenomation is made when the periocular erythema and edema are associated with an insect envenomation by history or by identification of a papular or vesicular lesion at the site of envenomation. Treatment is with cool compresses and antihistamines. Also give levofloxacin 500 mg once a day if secondary infection is suspected on the basis of increasing pain, redness, or swelling. Orbital cellulitis will also have periocular erythema and edema, but these signs will be accompanied by a history of sinusitis or upper respiratory tract infection, proptosis, restricted extraocular motility, decreased visual acuity, and/or fever. Orbital cellulitis is a life-threatening disorder and is treated with levofloxacin 500 mg twice a day, decongestants, and urgent evacuation.

C. Acute Red Eye

The differential diagnosis of the acute red eye includes both obvious and occult open globe injury, corneal abrasion or ulcer, subconjunctival hemorrhage, traumatic and nontraumatic iritis, hyphema, herpes simplex virus keratitis, corneal erosion, acute angle-closure glaucoma, scleritis, conjunctivitis, blepharitis, ultraviolet keratitis, episcleritis, conjunctival foreign body, dry eye, and contact lens overwear syndrome. A few simple diagnostic steps can be undertaken to help differentiate between the entities listed.

Wilderness Diagnostic Approach to Acute Red Eye

Trauma	No Trauma
Obvious open globe	Fluorescein test
Fluorescein test	Response to topical anesthesia
	Pupillary status

The first step is to inquire whether there has been recent trauma to the eye. If there has, the eye should be checked with a light source immediately to see if there is an obvious open globe. This type of injury is most often encountered in the presence of lacerating or impaling trauma, such as from a knife wound, a fishhook, or a tree branch or thorn impaling the globe. Should an obvious open globe be noted, immediately place a rigid shield (**not** a pressure patch) over the eye to protect it from further trauma. Start the victim immediately on levofloxacin 500 mg once daily and arrange for an urgent evacuation. Posttraumatic infection of the eye (called endophthalmitis) is a dreaded complication of an open globe and often results in permanent loss of vision.

If there is a history of eye trauma but no obvious open globe, perform a fluorescein stain with a fluorescein strip and a drop of topical anesthesia. Remove contact lenses prior to instilling the fluorescein stain. If an epithelial defect is seen with the cobalt blue light, the victim has either a corneal abrasion or a corneal ulcer. Several factors will help to differentiate the two. A corneal ulcer will often be seen as a white or gray spot on the cornea with a tangential penlight examination. No opacities or infiltrates are seen with a corneal abrasion. In addition, a corneal ulcer typically takes a day or two to develop after an episode of trauma and may be accompanied by a discharge. Increasing pain and photophobia are usually present with a developing corneal ulcer.

A traumatic corneal abrasion is treated with bacitracin ointment four times a day. Small or relatively less painful abrasions need not be patched. Diclofenac 0.1% drops four times a day may be added for pain control if needed. Sunglasses are helpful in reducing irritation from light if the eye is not patched. If the eye is patched because of a large or very painful abrasion, use bacitracin ointment before patching and recheck the eye in twenty-four hours. Scopolamine 0.25%, 1 drop bid or before patching, may be added for very painful abrasions but will result in blurring of near vision and a dilated pupil for three to six days. Systemic analgesics may also be required in some cases. Remove the patch daily to check for the development of a corneal ulcer and to repeat the fluorescein stain to monitor healing. Healing of the abrasion should occur within one to three days. If the trauma causing the abrasion is related to contact lens wear or insertion, there is a higher incidence of secondary infection with gram negative organisms and the eye should **not** be patched. Use topical ciprofloxacin four times a day until the abrasion is healed and watch the eye closely for development of a corneal ulcer.

If the diagnosis of corneal ulcer is made on the basis of trauma, an epithelial defect, and a white or gray spot on the cornea, treat with topical ciprofloxacin as follows: one drop every five minutes for three doses; one drop every fifteen minutes for six hours; then one drop every thirty minutes. Scopolamine 0.25% may be added for pain control if needed. A corneal ulcer is a vision-threatening disorder that may progress rapidly despite therapy, so evacuate urgently.

A posttraumatic red eye without an obvious open globe or an epithelial defect on fluorescein staining may represent a subconjunctival hemorrhage, traumatic iritis, hyphema, or an occult ruptured globe. A subconjunctival hemorrhage is a bright red area of blood overlying the sclera of the eye. It requires no treatment, but a careful inspection of the eye for associated injuries should be made. If the subconjunctival hemorrhage is massive and causes outward bulging of the conjunctiva (called chemosis), then suspect an occult ruptured globe and manage as described below.

Blood in the anterior chamber of the eye is called a hyphema. The primary concerns in this disorder are associated globe rupture and increased pressure in the eye. Urgently evacuate these individuals. Place a protective shield over the eye. Restrict activity to walking only. Do not let these individuals read. Do not treat them with NSAIDs or aspirin because of the increased risk of bleeding.

Traumatic iritis may follow blunt trauma to the globe or a corneal abrasion. Keys to diagnosis are pain and photophobia following blunt trauma or after a corneal abrasion has healed. Traumatic iritis typically resolves without treatment in several days, but severe cases may be treated with topical prednisolone 1% drops four times a day for three days. Although topical steroids should not generally be prescribed except by ophthalmologists, use of prednisolone drops will probably not cause any significant adverse effects if given to an individual with a fluorescein negative eye disorder for no more than three days.

Not all ruptured globes are obvious. An occult ruptured globe may be suspected on the basis of severe blunt trauma, a history of an impaling injury or one that results from metal-on-metal hammering, the presence of dark uveal tissue exposed at the limbus, a distorted pupil, or a decrease in vision. An occult ruptured globe also entails the possibility of endophthalmitis and is treated in the same manner as an obvious open globe.

If there is no history of trauma, the first important diagnostic step is a fluorescein stain. Should this test reveal an epithelial defect, the diagnostic possibilities include a corneal ulcer, a corneal erosion, or herpes simplex keratitis. The mechanism for corneal ulcer occurrence in the absence of a history of trauma is usually contact lens wear. Treat contact lens-related corneal ulcers as described for traumatic corneal ulcers except discontinue contact lens wear in **both** eyes immediately because the infection may be the result of contaminated lens solutions or cases.

The diagnosis of corneal erosion is made when there is an epithelial defect resembling a traumatic abrasion in the absence of a history of trauma. There is often a history of previous episodes. The onset of pain usually occurs when the eye is first opened in the morning. Treatment is as for a corneal abrasion.

Herpes simplex keratitis is diagnosed by a typical dendritic figure on fluorescein staining and the absence of a history of trauma. There is often a history of previous episodes. Urgently evacuate a patient with this finding.

If the fluorescein stain reveals no epithelial defect, the next useful bit of diagnostic information is the response of the eye pain to topical anesthesia. Relief of eye pain by topical anesthesia indicates that the pain is due to an ocular surface disease, some of which will be discussed below. If the pain is **not** significantly improved by topical anesthesia, then the next item of information needed is the size of the pupil in the affected eye compared to the fellow eye. If the pupil is dilated, then the likely diagnosis is angle-closure glaucoma (ACG). ACG usually occurs in patients over forty, is accompanied by a decrease in vision, and often by a history of previous episodes of eye pain. Treatment is with pilocarpine 2%, one drop every fifteen minutes times four doses in the affected eye, then four times a day in **both** eyes. Give acetazolamide 250 mg four times a day. Urgently evacuate the affected individual for definitive treatment with a laser iridotomy, since markedly elevated intraocular pressures may result in permanent damage to the optic nerve in twenty-four hours or less.

If the pain is **not** relieved by topical anesthesia, and the pupil is normal or constricted (miotic), then the likely diagnosis is either iritis or scleritis. Both diseases are often associated with systemic inflammatory disorders and may be vision threatening if not treated promptly and aggressively. Initiate treatment with prednisolone 1%, one drop every hour around the clock until evacuated. Also instill scopolamine 0.25%, one drop twice a day. The patient requires urgent evacuation. If improvement is not seen within twenty-four to forty-eight hours and evacuation has not been possible, start prednisone 80 mg once a day and continue until evacuation to definitive care is accomplished.

If the patient has no history of trauma, no epithelial defect or dendrites on fluorescein staining, and there is either no eye pain or the pain **is** significantly relieved by topical anesthesia, then the likely diagnosis is one of the disorders discussed below.

Conjunctivitis: Conjunctivitis is recognized by an acute onset, the presence of a discharge, exposure to other persons with eye infections, and/or URI symptoms. Treat with cipofloxacin one drop four times a day for five days. Caution the affected individual about possible spread of the infection to the other eye as well as to other individuals.

Blepharitis: This condition is often chronic with a history of previous exacerbations and remissions. It is more common in older individuals and is usually bilateral, although one eye may be more severely affected than the other. Treatment is with bacitracin ointment applied to the lid margins once a day at bedtime for three to four weeks. One week of four times a day application may be helpful in more severe cases. In addition, warm compresses used for ten minutes two to four times a day followed by gentle wiping away of the inflammatory material on the eyelashes is beneficial.

Keratitis: The diagnosis of UV keratitis, also known as snowblindness, is usually easy to make in the presence of bilateral eye pain and a sunburned face. As with sunburn of the skin, the symptoms do not reach their maximum intensity until several hours or longer after the exposure, so it is common for these patients to present in the evening hours. Fluorescein staining typically reveals no frank epithelial defect but numerous small dots of stain uptake called superficial punctate keratitis (SPK). Treatment is with bacitracin ointment four times a day until signs and symptoms resolve. These individuals are usually very photophobic and sunglasses are helpful. Patch severely affected eyes for comfort, although it is usually better to avoid patching both eyes if possible, for obvious reasons. Scopolamine 0.25%, one drop twice a day, may be helpful in relieving pain if the discomfort merits the blurred vision and dilated pupil that scopolamine therapy entails. Systemic analgesia may be required. Monitor these individuals daily until epithelial staining resolves to ensure that they do not develop a corneal ulcer.

Foreign material in eye: Although the abrupt onset of a foreign body sensation is strongly suggestive, definitive diagnosis requires identification of the foreign material, which may sometimes be quite difficult. Treatment consists of location and removal of the foreign body using enhanced lighting. Topical anesthesia will make the patient much more comfortable during the search and removal efforts. Use a hand-held magnifying lens or pair of reading glasses to aid in the examination. Eyelid eversion with a cotton-tipped applicator will help the examiner to identify foreign bodies located on the upper tarsal plate. Once located, remove the foreign body with a cotton-tipped applicator after the eye has been anesthetized and the cotton-tipped applicator moistened with tetracaine. The eye is then stained with fluorescein to check for a corneal abrasion. If no foreign body is visualized, but symptoms persist, vigorous irrigation with artificial tears or sweeps of the conjunctival fornices with a moistened cotton-tipped applicator after topical anesthesia may be successful in removing the foreign body.

Dry eye: Symptomatic dry eye is commonly encountered in the wilderness, especially in mountainous areas where the air is very dry and significant wind is often present. Dry eye is usually bilateral and may result in secondary tearing. There may be a history of previous episodes of symptomatic dry eye. Treatment is with artificial tears used as often as needed to relieve symptoms. Dehydration may contribute to this condition. The use of sunglasses may provide protection from the wind and be of significant benefit in managing this disorder.

Overwear syndrome: Contact lens overwear syndrome may be another source of ocular discomfort in the wilderness. The considerations here are much as described in the section above on dry eye, except that the symptoms are magnified by the presence of contact lenses. Contact lens rewetting drops and sunglasses are the first line of management. Should these measures be ineffective in relieving symptoms, remove the contact lenses. If significant SPK are present on fluorescein staining, use ciprofloxacin drops four times a day until the SPK have resolved. Do not replace contact lenses until the eye is symptom-free. An individual who wears contact lenses in the wilderness should **always** carry a pair of glasses that can be used if contact lens problems arise.

Episcleritis: Episcleritis is a generally benign and self-limited inflammation of the episclera (the lining of the eye between the conjunctiva and the sclera). There is usually sectoral redness without discharge and often a history of previous episodes. Discomfort is typically mild or absent. The presence of severe pain, photophobia, or decrease in vision suggests another diagnosis. Episcleritis is often misdiagnosed as conjunctivitis, but the lack of a discharge and the typical sectoral redness of episcleritis will help to differentiate between the two disorders. Episcleritis usually resolves without treatment over several weeks. If symptoms are troublesome, prednisolone 1% drops four times a day for three days may be used.

Subconjunctival hemorrhage: This condition may occur in the absence of trauma, often in association with coughing. Although the bright red appearance of the blood overlying the sclera may be alarming to the affected individual, this disorder is innocuous and will resolve without treatment over one to two weeks.

Chapter 10

HIGH-ALTITUDE ILLNESS

I. GENERAL INFORMATION

High-altitude illnesses affect large numbers of wilderness travelers and result in occasional deaths. The most common illnesses are acute mountain sickness (AMS), high-altitude pulmonary edema (HAPE), high-altitude cerebral edema (HACE), and peripheral edema. Proper management requires early diagnosis and prompt intervention. In the field, the safety of rescuers or the group may take precedence over ideal management of the patient.

II. GUIDELINES FOR PREVENTION

Most altitude illness is preventable. The following measures reduce the incidence and severity of high-altitude illness. Although these measures do not guarantee freedom from illness, they are highly recommended, especially for those without altitude experience.

A. Staged Ascent

Acclimatize by gradually increasing the altitude of overnight camps. If possible, the first camp should be no higher than 8,000 feet (2,400 meters), with an increase of no more than 1,000 to 2,000 feet (300 to 600 meters) per night. An alternative approach is to spend two nights at the same altitude for every 2,000-foot (600 meter) gain in altitude above 10,000 feet (3,000 meters). If a trip is started at over 9,000 feet (2,700 meters), two nights should be spent acclimatizing at that altitude before proceeding higher. Proceed higher during the day and return to a lower elevation to sleep (climb high, sleep low).

B. High-Carbohydrate Diet

A diet of at least 70 percent carbohydrates reduces symptoms of AMS by about 30 percent at altitudes above approximately 16,000 feet (5,000 meters) and can be started one to two days prior to ascent.

C. Appropriate Exercise Level

Until acclimatized, exercise moderately, avoiding excessive dyspnea and fatigue.

D. Hydration

To offset increased fluid losses at high altitudes, stay well hydrated. Adequate hydration may be judged by the presence of clear urine. It is, however, possible to overhydrate, which may worsen fluid retention with acute mountain sickness.

E. Drug Prophylaxis

Several drugs can lessen the symptoms of high-altitude illness. However, their use is not recommended as a routine measure.

1) Acetazolamide: The indications for acetazolamide prophylaxis are a forced rapid ascent, proceeding to sleeping altitude greater than 9,000 feet (2,700 meters) in one day from less than 4,000 feet (1,200 meters), or a history of previous AMS at similar rates of ascent. Acetazolamide reduces symptoms of AMS by about 75 percent. Acetazolamide is considered the drug of choice for chemoprophylaxis of AMS.

   The dose of acetazolamide for adults is 125 mg twice a day, starting the day of ascent. The dose for children is 5 mg/kg/day, up to the adult dose of 125 mg twice daily.

   Common side effects from this drug include peripheral paresthesia and polyuria. As this drug is a diuretic, the increase in urine fluid loss needs to be replaced. Contraindications are pregnancy, metabolic or respiratory acidosis, or allergy to sulfa drugs. Bone marrow suppression occurs, but is rare.

2) Dexamethasone: This drug can be used to prevent AMS either for those who cannot take acetazolamide, or for a forced rapid ascent to very high altitude, such as flying to over 14,000 feet (4,250 meters) on an overnight rescue.

   The dosage for adults is 4 mg orally every six to eight hours. Starting the medication two to four hours prior to ascent is probably adequate, although the exact timing for beginning and discontinuing the medication has not yet been established. Discontinuing dexamethasone before acclimatization has taken place may "unmask" the symptoms of AMS.

   Dyspepsia, bizarre dreams, dysphoria, and euphoria occasionally occur. The resulting lack of judgment in a dangerous mountain environment may have severe consequences.

3) Nifedipine: The prophylactic administration of nifedipine is effective in lowering pulmonary artery pressure and preventing high-altitude pulmonary edema in HAPE-susceptible individuals. The prophylactic dose of nifedipine is 30 or 60 mg (extended release formation) per day to be taken during the ascent phase of the expedition and for three additional days at altitude.

Possible side effects include dizziness, flushing or a feeling of warmth, headache, weakness, nausea, heartburn, muscle cramps, tremors, swelling of the arms or legs, nervousness, mood changes, low blood pressure, and heart palpitations. Long-term efficacy and the effects of withdrawal are not known. Consider the use of this drug for mountain sports only when the most important preventive measure, gradual ascent, has failed, and in patients with a previous history of HAPE.

F. Sedatives and Hypnotics

The use of sleeping medication increases the chance of developing symptoms of AMS. If a sleeping disorder is being complicated with periodic breathing (Cheyne-Stokes), the patient would probably benefit from acetazolamide use (see above) as opposed to sleeping medication.

III. GUIDELINES FOR ASSESSMENT AND TREATMENT

Ascending too quickly for an individual's physiology to cope with the hypoxic stress causes altitude illness. The treatment of choice for all forms of high-altitude illness is descent. However, mild forms of AMS usually resolve spontaneously in two to four days and descent is not necessary. There are few studies of treatment of AMS, and these guidelines reflect expert opinion more than well-controlled research studies. Treatment is based on four principles:

1) stop ascent in presence of symptoms (do not go up unless symptoms go away);
2) descend if there is no improvement or condition worsens;
3) descend immediately if HAPE, loss of coordination, or changes in level of consciousness are present;
4) ill persons must not be left alone or sent down alone.

HIGH-ALTITUDE ILLNESS

A. Acute Mountain Sickness

Individuals with AMS have headache, anorexia, nausea, insomnia, lack of normal diuresis, and lassitude. The syndrome resembles an alcohol hangover. There are no characteristic physical findings. Basic treatment is to descend or to stop ascent and wait for improvement before proceeding. Continuing ascent in the presence of symptoms is ill advised. After stopping the ascent, more advanced treatment consists of administering supplemental oxygen (1 L/min at rest), which is especially helpful during sleep. Aspirin or acetaminophen, with hydrocodone if necessary, is useful for headaches. Prochlorperazine or promethazine can be used for nausea. Prochlorperazine 10 mg parenterally or orally every six hours, or 25 mg rectally every twelve hours, for an average-size adult, also increases the hypoxic drive to breathe. Promethazine can be administered as 25 mg parenterally, or as 25 or 50 mg suppositories for adults every eight hours. Use no more than three doses of either drug. Note that both prochlorperazine and promethazine may cause extrapyramidal reactions requiring treatment with diphenhydramine. Treatment of the illness, rather than just the symptoms, requires acetazolamide. The treatment dose is 250 mg twice a day. Acetazolamide speeds acclimatization and aborts the illness. An alternative for persons who are sulfa allergic is dexamethasone (4 mg every six to eight hours). A response is usually seen within twelve to twenty-four hours. If the illness progresses, descent is mandatory.

B. High-Altitude Pulmonary Edema

Mild HAPE presents with decreased exercise performance, fatigue, dyspnea on exertion but not at rest, a dry cough, and localized rales. In moderate to severe HAPE there is marked weakness and fatigue, cyanosis, a dry to raspy cough, tachypnea, tachycardia, rales, a gurgling sensation in the chest, and, late in the course, a productive cough. Neurological symptoms and signs may also be present.

Oxygen, if available, improves arterial oxygenation and lowers pulmonary arterial pressure (PAP). Immediate descent is essential in moderate to severe cases with 2,000 to 4,000 feet (600 to 1,200 meters) usually being sufficient. Keep the patient warm and minimize exertion because both cold and exercise will raise the PAP.

Adjuncts to oxygen and descent may consist of nifedipine (20 mg stat sublingual, or chew and swallow, followed with 30 mg sustained release every six hours) in moderate to severe cases. An EPAP mask can be a temporizing measure. Even more important, a portable hyperbaric chamber (Gamow Bag) is highly useful in reversing the effects of high altitude when descent is impossible and can make a nonambulatory patient ambulatory. Constant monitoring of a patient in a Gamow Bag is mandatory. Length of time of treatment would be until symptoms cleared and the weather or climbing conditions permit the aided descent of the patient.

C. High-Altitude Cerebral Edema

Assessment of HACE is based on progressive neurological deterioration, with changes in consciousness or ataxia, progressing to impaired judgment, hallucinations, severe headache, and eventually coma. Basic treatment is immediate descent, until obvious improvement occurs, and/or a high flow of oxygen. With a pulse oximeter, give oxygen to achieve a saturation of 90 percent or greater. Be observant for concomitant HAPE. More advanced treatment includes dexamethasone eight to ten mg (by the route most easily achieved), followed by 4 mg every six hours until symptoms subside. Response is usually noted within twelve to twenty-four hours, but descent is still mandatory. Use the Gamow Bag, if it is available, as described above.

D. Peripheral Edema

High altitudes may cause swelling of the hands, ankles, or face (usually the periorbital region). Elevate the extremities, if possible. The edema will resolve with descent, but descent is not mandatory unless signs and symptoms of more serious altitude illnesses are present.

E. High Altitude Retinopathy

Retinal hemorrhages are common above 16,000 feet (5,000 meters), but may develop at lower altitudes. They are generally asymptomatic and do not warrant descent or other treatment. However, when a retinal hemorrhage overlies the macula it may cause blindness. They usually resolve after descent, although a blind spot may persist for years or permanently.

F. High Altitude Syncope

High altitude syncope is a benign entity that occurs at moderate altitudes. No treatment is necessary other than placing the patient supine or even in a slight head-down (Trendelenberg) position.

G. Splenic Infarction and Sickle Cell Crises

Splenic infarction, although rare, may occur as low as 5,000 feet (1,500 meters) in patients with sickle cell trait. Consider this condition as a possible cause of abdominal pain at altitude. Treatment of sickle cell crises is the same as at sea level.

Chapter 11

HYPOTHERMIA

I. GENERAL INFORMATION

Hypothermia occurs when the body's ability to generate and conserve heat is overcome by heat loss. **Acute** hypothermia presents with a sudden drop in body core temperature within a few hours. This is usually caused by immersion in cold water or a sudden drop in ambient temperature combined with wind and precipitation. **Chronic** hypothermia is the result of a gradual drop in body core temperature over several hours. Most chronic hypothermia deaths occur when the ambient temperature ranges from -1 to 10°C (30 to 50°F). Hypothermia is almost always preventable by minimizing heat loss via conduction, convection, radiation, and evaporation. Prevention includes 1) proper choice and use of clothing and shelter; 2) avoidance of overexertion; 3) staying dry (a combination of proper clothing and avoidance of overexertion); 4) staying well hydrated; and 5) maintenance of adequate nutrition.

A. Mild Hypothermia

Hypothermia is considered mild if the core temperature is below 35°C (95°F) and above 32°C (90°F). In this temperature range, the thermoregulatory defense mechanisms, such as shivering, are generally unimpaired and operating maximally. Mild hypothermia often first manifests itself as loss of judgment and fine motor coordination. Shivering is often suppressed by physical activity, but by the time core temperature reaches 35°C (95°F), most patients are shivering uncontrollably. Vigorous shivering will be seen during further cooling to 32°C (90°F), except in some chronic exposure situations (more than six to eight hours) where exhaustion and shivering fatigue may occur. Slurred speech, a stumbling gait, and the development of ataxia are highly suggestive of hypothermia in a cold-exposed patient. It is important to note that most patients with mild hypothermia are fully able to rewarm themselves through shivering heat production, although they require protection from further heat loss in order to do so. The exception will be an exhausted patient who is unable to shiver.

B. Moderate-to-Severe Hypothermia

Hypothermia is considered moderate at core temperatures below 32°C (90°F) and above 28°C (82°F), and severe at core temperatures below 28°C (82°F).

Since taking rectal temperatures may not be possible or appropriate, diagnosis can be based on observations and functional characteristics.

As core temperature decreases within the moderate range, thermoregulatory shivering is progressively inhibited until it stops and the patient loses the ability to rewarm (usually at a core temperature of about 30°C (86°F). The patient may have a profoundly altered mental status, loss of coordination, lassitude, and an apathetic attitude. Finally, consciousness will be lost.

As core temperature decreases below 28°C (82°F) (severe hypothermia), the heart is at risk of ventricular fibrillation either spontaneously due to low heart temperature, or as a reflex response to mechanical stimulation. The patient is consciousness and pupils may be dilated and fixed. The torso will be cold to touch. The patient may be rigid and unresponsive, with nonpalpable pulse and respirations, but not dead (the patient cannot be presumed dead unless these conditions persist after warming).

II. GUIDELINES FOR FIELD TREATMENT

A. General Principles

The general principles of treatment apply for all cases of hypothermia. The patient must be gently removed from the cold exposure and must remain in a horizontal position. Remove wet clothing carefully and insulate the patient with special attention given to the head and neck (i.e., with one or even two sleeping bags if possible). This will minimize convective and conductive heat loss. A vapor barrier (i.e., plastic sheet or space blanket) can be added around other insulation to eliminate evaporative heat loss.

B. Mild Hypothermia

A mildly hypothermic patient will be shivering vigorously and may be dehydrated. Administer fuel for shivering with warm high-energy drinks (nonalcohol) and foods, providing the patient is alert and can swallow without choking.

External heat sources such as chemical or charcoal heat packs and hot water bottles can be used. For rewarming purposes, the heat should be applied preferentially to the chest, armpits, and neck with additional sources to the groin, if available. During winter transport heat should be applied to the soles of the feet to prevent frostbite (provided frostbite is not already present). Place the palms of the hands on the chest heat source. Do not apply these heat sources directly to the patient's skin, but wrap them in clothing. A patient may also be placed in two sleeping bags zipped together with one to two dry normothermic rescuers. This will be unlikely to enhance the rewarming rate of a vigorously shivering patient but may provide some psychological support. Before initiating body-to-body rewarming, these factors should be weighed against personnel and equipment implications and the difficulty of evacuation of two to three persons together.

Exercise will generate heat but may also precipitate a significant drop in core temperature (afterdrop). If the patient is otherwise healthy and vigorously shivering, mild exercise may be initiated only after forty-five to sixty minutes of shivering in an insulated environment. At this point the afterdrop should be reversed. However, if any deterioration in physical or mental condition occurs during exercise, it should stop immediately.

C. Moderate-to-Severe Hypothermia

Whether a patient is moderately or severely hypothermic, the clinical condition is serious: treatment is the same **under all circumstances**. The patient must be handled very gently and kept in the horizontal position. Because of the risk of inducing ventricular fibrillation, remove wet clothing and take care to minimize patient movement while performing other life-sustaining measures. Make arrangements to transfer the patient to medical facilities as soon as possible.

Shivering will be weak, intermittent or nonexistent, and the patient will not warm up spontaneously. The condition may degenerate progressively. Application of moderate heat to the skin is indicated. Place external heat sources, such as heat packs, inside the barrier as indicated above. Body-to-body contact with one or two rescuers may provide a warming advantage in this condition.

Warmed and humidified supplemental oxygen may be administered. This is unlikely to significantly heat the body core; however, improvement in cardiovascular and mental function has been reported with this treatment.

Do not give a patient with impaired consciousness any warm drinks as they may cause burns and/or choking. Aggressive rewarming, such as warm water immersion, may also cause ventricular fibrillation. Do not rub the extremities.

D. Cardiopulmonary Resuscitation

Do not initiate CPR in patients with greatly diminished yet viable cardiac output. Such action may initiate ventricular fibrillation. Respiration and pulse may be slow, shallow, and difficult to detect. Therefore, rescuers should take forty-five to sixty seconds to carefully assess these vital signs. If neither pulse nor breath is detected, CPR should be initiated in accordance with normal, basic life support protocols.

III. GUIDELINES FOR EVACUATION

Once a patient with mild hypothermia is adequately rewarmed, with a return to normal mental status, there is no need for evacuation. Take care to prevent a recurrence. Monitor the patient while walking with him/her to the nearest location where treatment is practical. Patients who do not respond to rewarming, or who obviously have moderate-to-severe hypothermia, must be insulated for maximum heat retention, provided with moderate heat source(s), and be evacuated as soon as possible. Evacuation of such a patient must be as gentle as possible to prevent ventricular fibrillation. Package the person so that rescue personnel are able to examine the patient periodically. Every fifteen minutes during transport check the patient for vital signs, burning of the skin underneath heat sources, and check circulation in the feet to look for frostbite.

Chapter 12

FROSTBITE AND IMMERSION FOOT

I. GENERAL INFORMATION

Frostbite is localized injury or death of tissue due to freezing of cells. The chance of damage is increased by: 1) temperatures below -2°C (28°F), and especially temperatures of -7°C (20°F) or less; 2) high winds and/or high altitude; 3) use of tobacco, alcohol, or other drugs; 4) contact with heat-conductive materials such as metal, water, or gasoline; 5) overexertion, which produces fatigue and sweat, and; 6) previous frostbite injury.

Measures to help prevent frostbite include: 1) minimizing direct exposure of skin to cold environment; 2) avoiding tight boots or too many pairs of socks in larger boots; 3) preserving heat by keeping head, neck, and face covered; 4) wearing mittens instead of gloves; 5) staying well hydrated; 6) maintaining metabolic heat production with adequate caloric intake; 7) keeping dry; and 8) avoiding direct skin-metal or skin-fluid contact.

Immersion foot (trenchfoot) is a cold weather, nonfreezing injury resulting from prolonged exposure to a cold, wet environment. The primary injuries are vasoconstriction of the arterioles with subsequent loss of heat and oxygen supply to surface tissues and damage to peripheral nerves. Prevention includes: 1) avoidance of tight-fitting footwear; 2) changing into dry socks regularly (at least once a day); and 3) periodic (every 4 hours in extreme wet and cold conditions) air drying, elevation, and massaging of feet to promote circulation.

II. GUIDELINES FOR ASSESSMENT AND TREATMENT

A. Superficial frostbite (frostnip)

A small patch of skin is white but rapidly returns to normal with warm breath or skin-to-skin rewarming. No special treatment required.

B. Partial thickness frostbite

The skin is pale, cold, and numb, but underlying tissues remain soft and pliable. Treat superficial frostbite with passive skin-to-skin contact or rapid rewarming, but avoid heat exposure greater than 42°C (108°F). After thawing, a few clear fluid-filled blisters develop in superficial frostbite. If damage is extensive, blisters may fill with bloody fluid, and treatment should be administered as in deep frostbite (see below). Extreme care must be taken with frostbitten tissue to prevent refreezing. Evacuate as soon as possible if blisters have formed. This can be a self-evacuation if the hands are involved but might require a litter evacuation if the feet are affected. If possible give ibuprofen before spontaneous or therapeutic thawing. Maintain adequate hydration. Treat topically with aloe vera; otherwise, manage as for a superficial burn.

C. Full thickness (deep) frostbite

Skin and deep structures, including muscle, tendons, and possibly even bone are involved. The affected part is hard and not pliable. On diagnosis of deep frostbite, evacuate patient immediately. Patients with frostbitten, unthawed feet may walk to self-evacuate. During evacuation, if possible, protect the affected part with dry insulation, such as clean dry socks or dry mittens. Remove jewelry and all constrictive clothing. After evacuation, or if transportation is certain, rapidly rewarm the frostbitten area in water preheated to 40 to 42°C (104 to 108°F). Suspend the frostbitten area in the container of water without allowing contact with the sides. Check water temperature often to maintain the temperature at 37 to 40°C (99 to 104°F). Avoid excessive heat as this increases the pain and cellular damage. During thawing, pain is usually severe and analgesics, including narcotics, are indicated. After thawing, multiple fluid-filled and hemorrhagic blisters form. The portion of the extremity beyond the hemorrhagic blisters is extremely damaged and may eventually become gangrenous. When rewarming is accomplished, dry the affected parts gently, place sterile gauze between digits, and apply aloe vera or antibiotic ointment gently to damaged skin. Elevate the injured part. Give 400 mg of ibuprofen before rewarming and every six hours to inhibit thromboxane production, which causes increased cellular damage. Maintain adequate hydration. Provide definitive medical care as soon as possible.

D. Immersion foot

Injury includes cold, swollen, waxy feet, mottled with dark burgundy to blue splotches. Skin is sodden and friable. In the later stage, feet become red, hot, and very painful. Blisters often form. Infection and gangrene frequently result. Field treatment includes 1) maintenance of dry, warm feet; 2) oral hydration; 3) ibuprofen every six hours to inhibit thromboxane production; and 4) immediate evacuation to definitive care (note: walking may be difficult for the patient).

III. CONTROVERSIES

A. Should deep frostbite be thawed in the field? There is evidence that the longer tissue stays frozen, the worse the injury. Frozen extremities in an otherwise uninjured patient are difficult to keep frozen, and spontaneous thawing usually occurs during evacuation. Field therapy, which can render an ambulatory patient nonambulatory, must be balanced against the time required for evacuation.

B. Should a patient self-evacuate on frozen toes/feet prior to thawing if worse freezing is unlikely or field thawing can not be easily accomplished? The longer the extremity is frozen, the greater the tissue damage, although even more significant damage occurs with a thaw followed by freezing. The decision to walk out on frozen feet should not be made if there is any reasonable ability to thaw and provide further protection from freezing. Thawed toes may not be so painful as to preclude self-evacuation. Deep frostbite of the entire foot may become so painful and debilitating upon thawing that self-evacuation becomes impossible. As field assessment of severity may be difficult before thawing, frozen extremities should generally be thawed and protected from further freezing as soon as possible, realizing that the victim might not be able to self-evacuate.

Chapter 13

HEAT-RELATED ILLNESSES

I. GENERAL INFORMATION

Heat-related illnesses comprise several conditions, caused by exposure to hot environments, or intense exercise in moderate environments that range from mild discomfort to life-threatening illness. Hyperthermia occurs when heat stress on the body, from internal metabolic heat production and external sources, overcomes the body's heat dissipating. Extreme untreated hyperthermia can rapidly become life threatening.

Heat illnesses are preventable. Prevention includes:

1) Acclimatization, the process by which the body adapts to heat exposure, is induced by a minimum of sixty to ninety minutes of exercise in the heat each day for one to two weeks. Initial adaptation occurs within a few days. The most significant change is an increase in sweat volume initiated at a lower skin temperature. This increases evaporative cooling and results in a lower heart rate and core temperature for a given amount of work in the heat.

2) Hydration with adequate fluid quantities. An acclimatized person can lose one liter (two pints) per hour of sweat during exercise. Relieving thirst alone risks not maintaining full hydration. Start each work period by drinking 500 ml (approximately one pint) of water. At least 300 to 500 ml per hour is then likely to be required, and requirements may be higher with extreme exertion or sweat loss (see Oral Fluid and Electrolyte Replacement).

3) Dress appropriately in light-colored, loose-fitting clothing, allowing maximum evaporative heat loss.

4) Frequent rest, especially before full acclimatization, preferably in shade, and ideally with a wipe of cool water on exposed areas of skin.

5) Maximize evaporative cooling by dipping clothing periodically in water, if possible.

6) Physical fitness improves the rate and quality of acclimatization, but does not provide heat adaptation by itself. The insulation of excess body fat reduces heat loss.

II. GUIDELINES FOR ASSESSMENT AND TREATMENT

A. Heat cramps

These muscle spasms may be severe, and are usually in large, heavily exercised muscle groups like legs and abdomen. They are probably caused by a combination of electrolyte depletion, hyperventilation with respiratory alkalosis, and plasma volume depletion. Rest the patient and give oral or intravenous fluids that contain sodium. Cold oral fluids are absorbed more quickly than warm ones. Gentle massaging of the cramped muscles is usually beneficial. After recovery, the activity may be resumed, but if the cramps return, a twenty-four-hour rest is recommended.

B. Heat syncope

Seen immediately after periods of strenuous work in hot environments. Patients regain consciousness quickly. Treat with recumbent rest in a cooler area and splash water on exposed skin, to enhance cooling. Oral rehydration is indicated when the patient is fully alert. Assess the patient for injuries if a fall was associated with the syncope.

C. Heat rash

Also called prickly heat, or miliaria, this acute inflammatory disease of the skin is seen in humid regions following prolonged sweating. Sweat gland ducts become blocked with keratinizing cells and accumulated sweat is forced through the duct walls, inciting inflammation in adjacent soft tissue. Erythematous pruritic papules appear on trunk and extremities, excluding hands and feet. Secondary infection may occur. In severe cases heat tolerance is reduced due to decreased sweating. In the field, keep the affected areas clean and limit exercise and heat exposure.

D. Heat exhaustion

Caused by dehydration and intravascular volume depletion in a thermally stressful environment. Symptoms and signs include: weakness, inability to work, headache, mild confusion, nausea, faintness, anorexia, dyspnea, and rapid pulse. Skin may be warm or cool with sweating. The core temperature may be normal or moderately elevated. In practice, the distinction between heat exhaustion and heat stroke may be somewhat blurred. Should doubt exist, always err on the side of caution and treat as for heat stroke (see below). Otherwise remove the patient to a cooler area, allow him/her to rest, and rehydrate orally, preferably with cold, lightly-salted water or an electrolyte solution. The patient may benefit from cooling of the skin by wetting and fanning. When the patient has fully recovered, the activity may continue. Depending on the extent of the illness, recovery may take as long as twenty-four hours.

E. Heat stroke

This is a true medical emergency in which elevated core body temperature (above 40.5°C [105°F], rectally) causes renal, hepatic, and nervous system damage. Persons at increased risk of heat stroke include those who are obese, unfit, unacclimatized, elderly, acutely ill, dehydrated from vomiting or diarrhea; individuals with underlying medical conditions such as coronary heart disease and hyperthyroidism; and individuals on certain medications, e.g., beta-blockers, stimulants, diuretics, or anticholinergics.

Skin may be dry or sweating may be intact, especially in a fit person suffering exertional heat stroke. Symptoms and signs include confusion, disorientation, bizarre behavior, ataxia, tachycardia, tachypnea, and hot, red skin. Both heat stroke and heat exhaustion may present as collapse in the face of a heat load—environmental heat, metabolic heat from exercise, or a combination of both. Both may have altered consciousness, elevated temperatures, and rapid pulse. Heat stroke is differentiated from heat exhaustion by the presence of cardiovascular shock, persistent profound mental status changes, and markedly elevated temperature. In heat exhaustion, mental status and blood pressure normalize rapidly as in syncope, if the patient is recumbent in the shade.

Heat stroke has a high mortality rate. Whenever there is altered mental status and elevated temperature, rapid cooling is essential and must be started in the field. Treatment may include: 1) shading from direct sunlight and removal of clothing; 2) spraying with tepid or cool water and fanning aggressively; 3) ice packs at the neck, armpits, and groin; and 4) massage of extremities to return cooler peripheral blood to the core.

If possible, check the rectal temperature every 5 to 10 minutes and, when the temperature reaches approximately 37.7 to 38.8°C (100 to 102°F), taper off the cooling efforts, as rapid cooling below this point may lead to shivering. If the patient returns to a level of consciousness appropriate for oral hydration, give fluids. Do not give antipyretics like aspirin or acetaminophen. Rapid evacuation is indicated. Monitor carefully for rebound temperature increase.

Chapter 14

LIGHTNING INJURIES

I. GENERAL INFORMATION

One bolt of lightning may generate 300,000 amps and 2 billion volts—an awesome power capable of great destructive force. A single strike often injures or kills more than one person. Lightning injures or kills in one of four ways: 1) direct strike; 2) splash after striking a nearby object; 3) ground current; or 4) trauma from the blast of exploding air. Lightning causes serious injury or death in about one-third of its victims and permanent sequelae of some sort in about two-thirds of survivors. The factors related to a fatal outcome include immediate cardiopulmonary arrest or the presence of leg or head burns. Because any electrical current takes the shortest path between contact points, leg or head burns may mean that multiple organ systems have been injured. The duration of a lightning strike is so brief (less than one millisecond) that it may not penetrate but "flash over" the patient's skin.

Although lightning strikes are unpredictable, there are ways to reduce the chance of injury. During an electrical storm: 1) avoid open areas where you are one of the tallest objects, 2) do not seek shelter under a single tree, bush, or rock that stands in an open area, 3) avoid extremes of high or low ground, 4) avoid contact with metal objects unless you can get completely inside of one (such as an enclosed automobile), 5) seek shelter deep in a dry cave, staying away from the sides and roof, 6) seek shelter among trees or bushes or rocks of uniform size, 7) if boating, attempt to get to shore, waves and shoreline permitting, 8) squat with your feet close together or sit in a compact position on a nonconductive material, such as a foam pad or rope coil, and 9) spread out a group but stay close enough to maintain visual contact with each other.

II. GUIDELINES FOR ASSESSMENT

Victims of lightning strike are not electrically charged and pose no threat to rescuers. Patients typically fall into one of three categories: 1) minimally injured, requiring little immediate care other than psychological support, although they must receive a thorough examination when time allows, 2) seriously injured, often initially unconscious, requiring immediate attention to airway and obvious injuries, including appropriate stabilization for possible head and spine injuries, and 3) maximally injured, in cardiopulmonary arrest, requiring long-term efforts at CPR, which may result in full recovery. Fixed, dilated pupils may be a transient phenomenon.

With multiple casualties, unlike normal triage situations, give priority care to those who appear dead after a lightning strike. These victims may be salvaged by prolonged CPR. Evacuate all patients surviving a lightning strike for definitive medical evaluation and treatment.

For patients who are not in cardiac arrest but who are unconscious, consider placing a controlled airway (naso- or endotracheal tube, or cricothyrotomy). Therapy for increased intracranial pressure (see Head Injury, Chapter 4 and Spinal Injury, Chapter 5) may be necessary.

In patients with cardiac arrest, continue CPR. Investigate for multiple-organ injuries, including cardiac, renal, and CNS injury.

Promptly investigate the hypotensive patient for major hemorrhage, spinal shock, or fluid loss from burns. Internal burns of muscles may result in extensive fluid loss, out of proportion to the external burns. Test vision and hearing. Assess and advise the patient that tetanus immunization must be current. Admit patients with major injuries, arrhythmias, altered mental status, neurological changes, or chest pain to the hospital. Reexamine all patients within twenty-four hours and advise of the potential for immediate and delayed sequelae, including neurological, renal, cardiac, and muscular dysfunction.

Chapter 15

FIELD WATER DISINFECTION

I. GENERAL INFORMATION

Wilderness surface water carries a risk of enteric illness due to ingestion of waterborne pathogens that include bacteria, viruses, protozoan cysts, and some parasitic eggs or larvae. Risk varies with geographic location. In North America, *Giardia lamblia* is the most common microbial contaminant, but *Campylobacter jejuni,* enterotoxigenic *E. coli,* enteric viruses, and *Cryptosporidium* have caused outbreaks of illness. In developing countries, surface and tap water must be considered contaminated. Potential microorganisms include protozoa (*Entamoeba histolytica, Giardia lamblia, Cryptosporidium*), bacteria (*E. coli, Shigella, Vibrio cholerae, Salmonella, C. jejuni, V. parahaemolyticus*), viruses (hepatitis A and other enteric viruses), or helminths. Potable drinking water can be prepared by disinfecting water using one of several means.

II. METHODS OF WATER DISINFECTION

A. Heat

As in pasteurization, temperatures above 70°C (160°F) kill all enteric pathogens within thirty minutes, and 85°C (185°F) is effective within a few minutes. Thus, disinfection occurs during the time required to heat water from 60°C (140°F) to boiling temperature, so any water brought to a boil, even at high altitudes, is safe.

B. Filtration

This may be used for *Giardia* and other protozoal cysts, enteric bacteria, and parasitic eggs. However, for field use, filtration alone does not adequately remove viruses, although many are removed by adhering to larger particles. The maximum effective filter pore size for *Giardia* and amoeba cysts is 5 microns. For enteric bacteria, it is 0.2 to 0.5 microns, depending on filter design. *Cryptosporidium* oocysts require less than 3 microns pore size, while other parasitic eggs and larvae are removed with a 20 to 30 micron filter. Most commercial filters claim removal of *Giardia* only or *Giardia* and bacteria. Claims for viral removal should be discounted because they are not well substantiated. Some filters incorporate activated charcoal or an iodine resin. (See techniques below.)

C. Clarification techniques

These remove suspended particulate matter and many microorganisms. They are not adequate to disinfect water reliably but may be used to improve clarity and remove organic matter prior to filtration or halogenation.

1) Sedimentation is the separation of large particles by gravity. Simply allow water to stand in any container for at least one hour and then decant.

2) Coagulation, flocculation (C-F) removes smaller, suspended particles (colloids) that will not settle with simple gravity. This method works best on "cloudy" water, such as brown or green water that is loaded with organic material, as opposed to inorganic matter such as fine clay particles. Add alum (aluminum sulfate) to water (⅛ to ¼ tsp/gal) and mixed thoroughly. Then stir or gently agitate occasionally for five minutes and allow to settle. Colloidal particles clump together and then settle by gravity or float. The clear water can be decanted, filtered or poured through a cloth or coffee filter. The majority of microorganisms will settle with the floc, but a second disinfection step is recommended. Alum can be obtained at chemical supply stores or some grocery stores (pickling powder). If alum is not available, lime or the fine white ash from a campfire can be used.

3) Charcoal filters (purifiers) alone are not adequate for disinfection, although they improve the taste and appearance of water by absorbing chemicals.

D. Halogens

Chlorine and iodine are effective disinfectants for viruses, bacteria, and protozoan cysts (excluding *Cryptosporidium*). Both are available in tablet or liquid form. Iodine also comes in crystalline or polymolecular resin form. In equivalent concentrations, iodine has some advantages over chlorine for field use, less reactivity with organic matter, and less sensitivity to pH.

The effectiveness of a halogen depends on its concentration, the temperature of the water, and the amount of time it is left in the water (contact time). Weaker concentrations or colder water necessitate longer contact time. In the wilderness, the residual concentration cannot be measured, so some uncertainty results. Very high doses of halogen may be used to overcome the uncertainty, but this results in unacceptable taste. Smaller doses are effective in clean water if a prolonged contact time is used. Detection of a faint halogen color, smell, or taste indicates the presence of residual halogen in the water.

Because iodine and chlorine react with organic impurities to form a relatively inactive compound, the dose must be increased in grossly contaminated or cloudy water. Inorganic particulate matter does not react with halogens but can be removed by straining, filtering, sedimentation, or coagulation to improve taste. It is best to clarify water before treatment with halogens. Palatable surface water has a nearly neutral pH, which is optimal for effective treatment with a halogen.

Taste may be improved by several means:

1) Decrease the amount of halogen while increasing contact time

2) Add flavored drink mix after adequate contact time

3) Pour water through a charcoal filter after adequate contact time

4) Use techniques that do not leave residual halogen, such as heat or filters

5) Remove the halogen taste by using a zinc brush (see page 64), sodium thiosulfate, ascorbic acid (vitamin C), or hydrogen peroxide in combination with calcium hypochlorite (see page 64)

An alternative to iodine should be sought for pregnant women (although the amount ingested from a filter with an iodine resin is safe). Caution should be exercised if iodine is used for more than two weeks with anyone on lithium (establish stable medication dose and confirm normal thyroid function) or with an active thyroid disease.

Disinfection Techniques and Halogen Doses

(All doses added to one quart water: dose/contact time)

Iodination techniques	amount for 4 ppm	amount for 8 ppm
Iodine tabs	½ tab	1 tab
tetraglycine hydroperiodide		
EDWGT (emergency		
drinking water germicidal tablet)		
Potable Aqua		
Globaline		
2% iodine solution (tincture)	0.2 ml	0.4 ml
	5 gtts	10 gtts
10% povidone-iodine solution	0.35 ml	0.70 ml
	8 gtts	16 gtts
Saturated iodine crystals in water		
(commercial name: Polar Pure)	13 ml	26 ml
Saturated iodine crystals in alcohol	0.1 ml	0.2 ml
	amount for 5 ppm	amount for 10 ppm
Halazone tabs		
mono-dichloraminobenzoic acid	2 tabs	4 tabs
Household bleach 5%	0.1 ml	0.2 ml
Sodium hypochlorite	2 gtts	4 gtts

Concentration of halogenon	Contact time in minutes at various water temperaturess		
	5°C/41°F	15°C/59°F	30°C/86°F
2 ppm	240	180	60
4 ppm	180	60	45
8 ppm	60	30	15

Note: Recent data indicate that very cold water requires prolonged contact time with iodine or chlorine to kill *Giardia* cysts. These contact times in cold water have been extended from the usual recommendations to account for this and for the uncertainty of residual concentration.

III. TECHNIQUES FOR WATER DISINFECTION

A. Iodine resins

The resin releases iodine on contact that binds to microorganisms. The exact mechanism of iodine transfer to organisms is not known. Minimal iodine dissolves in water: effluent contains 0.5 to 2.0 ppm iodine. This dissolved iodine is not responsible for disinfection, so many filters include a charcoal resin to remove all iodine dissolved in the water after passing through the iodine resin. Some devices incorporate a 1 micron filter to remove cysts that are resistant to iodine (*Cryptosporidium*) or require longer contact times (*Giardia*). Potential problems include channeling of water through the resin, which may allow some organisms through without contacting the iodine resin.

B. Chlorination-dechlorination

This technique uses very high concentrations of chlorine for disinfection, then "dechlorination" with peroxide, which forms soluble calcium chloride, a tasteless and odorless compound. Excess peroxide bubbles off as oxygen. The kit consists of chlorine crystals (calcium hypochloride) and 30% hydrogen peroxide in separate small Nalgene bottles. This is a very good technique for highly polluted or cloudy waters, for disinfecting large volumes, and for storing water on boats. *Note:* 30% peroxide is extremely corrosive and burns skin.

C. Flocculation-chlorination

Tablets contain both alum for a flocculent and chlorine for a disinfectant. This has the advantage of cleaning and disinfecting cloudy or foul smelling water in a one-step process. The tablet is designed to leave 8 ppm free residual chlorine after flocculation, but 3 to 5 ppm is more common. Extend the recommended fifteen minute contact time for added safety in cold water.

D. Dehalogenation

A small wand with brush-like zinc and copper alloy bristles is used to stir the water to dechlorinate. It is intended to be used after halogenation. Zinc catalyzes an electrochemical reaction reducing hypochlorite to chloride or iodine to iodide, neither of which has taste, smell, or color. Zinc is not used up so the life span of the product is indefinite. The device is practical only for small amounts of water at a time. Larger volumes or higher concentrations require a considerable amount of time. Very small amounts of sodium thiosulfate or ascorbic acid will accomplish the same chemical reduction, removing halogen taste. These techniques should be used only after adequate contact time.

IV. CONTROVERSIES

A. What is the best technique? The best technique depends on personal preference and intended use. Use of heat may be limited by fuel supplies. If planned for a large group, halogenation or high-capacity filters work best. Two-stage techniques are more effective as water quality deteriorates.

Iodine and chlorine have similar antimicrobial activity, although there may be some advantages to iodine. Most prefer the taste of iodine over chlorine in equipotent doses, and iodine is less reactive with nitrogenous wastes in the water. However, iodine is physiologically active, and may be unsafe for individuals with iodine allergies, for those with uncontrolled thyroid disease, and for prolonged use in pregnant women. Although not proven dangerous in healthy individuals, iodine use should be limited to months, not years.

Filtration is not a reliable method for removing viruses. Although viral contamination is currently unlikely in North American alpine surface water, high levels of viral contamination should be assumed in lowland rivers with towns upstream and in developing countries. In these areas, halogenation or heat should be used instead of, or in addition to, filtration.

B. Is *Cryptosporidium* a sufficient risk to mandate filtration of surface water? *Cryptosporidium* is a protozoan, transmitted by the fecal-oral route, that can cause enteric illness. It produces a hardy oocyst. Waterborne outbreaks have been demonstrated and the oocysts have been found to be widespread in surface water. Although pathogenicity is not debated, the epidemiology of infection, specifically the incidence of symptomatic infection and presence of immunity, is unclear. The problem is that the oocyst is extremely resistant to halogens.

C. Are waterborne pathogens a significant source of illness for wilderness and foreign travelers? The major source of traveler's diarrhea is food borne. However, waterborne outbreaks of most enteric pathogens have been confirmed, and the waterborne route has been shown to be a major source of giardiasis outbreaks in the United States, especially from surface water. While the risk of illness from wilderness water in North America may be small and considered negligible by some, countries without sanitation have a much higher risk due to high levels of enteric pathogens in surface water.

Chapter 16

ORAL FLUID AND ELECTROLYTE REPLACEMENT

I. GENERAL INFORMATION

Oral rehydration/electrolyte solutions (ORS) are useful in three circumstances when fluids and electrolytes may be lost in significant amounts: 1) heavy, prolonged exercise with high-volume sweat losses; 2) treatment of mild to moderate heat illness; and 3) illness with diarrhea and/or vomiting. Significant hemorrhage also requires fluid replacement.

A. Fluid replacement during exercise

Large fluid losses may occur during exercise in heat and at high altitudes. Sweat losses of one liter (two pints) per hour are common during moderate exercise in a hot environment or at high levels of exertion in a temperate environment. The rate is individual and depends on the degree of heat acclimatization. Dehydration disposes to heat illness. In high altitude mountaineering, the scarcity of surface water, difficulty adjusting clothing to changing levels of exertion or weather conditions, and respiratory fluid losses from hyperventilation in dry, cold air commonly create fluid needs of seven to eight liters (approximately two gallons) per day. Dehydration in this environment disposes to altitude sickness, hypothermia, frostbite, and venous thrombosis.

During exercise, fluid replacement is critical. Inadequate fluid intake decreases performance and increases the risk of heat illness. Too much fluid may lead to dilutional hyponatremia. For most situations, at least 300 to 500 mls (approximately one pint) per hour will be required. Needs will be higher with extreme exertion or environment. The fluid is best consumed in volumes of approximately 200 mls (one-half pint) at a time as this promotes emptying of the stomach. Dark urine suggests that the body is struggling to maintain normal hydration and can be used as a sign that fluid intake should be increased.

Sweat contains electrolytes: sodium (average 20 to 60 mEq/L), chloride, and small amounts of potassium. In most instances, replacement of electrolytes during sweat loss is not necessary, so ORS have no advantage over plain water. Electrolyte needs can usually be met by regular meals and snacks, which also provide more calories than electrolyte solutions.

In endurance events or work/exercise for more than two hours in a very hot environment with high sweat losses, electrolyte supplements are recommended. During exercise, a solution containing 2 to 6% glucose and 30 mEq/L sodium is optimal to maintain palatability. Higher glucose concentrations may delay gastric emptying and promote osmotic diarrhea, but new long-chain carbohydrates that break down to simple sugars during digestion can provide larger amounts of sugar. Excessive sodium can cause nausea. Do not ingest salt tablets directly because they can cause gastric irritation and vomiting. One or two salt tablets, however, can be dissolved in a liter of water.

Commercial sports drinks contain about 6% glucose and 10 to 25 mEq/L of sodium. Simple solutions can be made at home. One teaspoon sugar in one liter (approximately one quart) of water yields a 0.35 to 0.5% solution, so three to four tsp sugar in a liter yields a 1 to 2% solution with about 50 kcal. One-half tsp NaCl (table salt) added to 1 liter of water yields about 30 mEq/L. In the wilderness, it is convenient to replace salt with snack foods during exertion. Although the teaspoon measurement method is quite variable (yielding 3.5 to 5.0 cc), concentrations over the resulting range are not dangerous.

B. Treatment of mild heat illness

Oral electrolyte solutions are an excellent means of treating mild to moderate forms of heat illness such as heat syncope, heat cramps, and heat exhaustion. The patient must rest in the shade and sip fluids. Usually 1 to 2 liters (two to four pints) of fluids similar to exercise replacement fluids are adequate. Oral fluids cannot be used for heat stroke, during altered consciousness, unless via a nasogastric tube. There is an increased risk of aspiration with a nasogastric tube if the patient is comatose or has a seizure.

C. Replacement of enteric fluid losses

Diarrheal illness (e.g., traveler's diarrhea) is the main indication for oral electrolyte solutions. Most cases of infectious enteritis are self-limited, although antibiotics can shorten the duration of most bacterial enteric infections. The major morbidity from these infections results from dehydration, so rehydration and maintenance of fluids and electrolytes are essential. Diarrheal fluid contains more electrolytes than sweat: sodium (50 to 100 mEq/L), chloride, and significant amounts of potassium and bicarbonate. Oral replacement is feasible because the gut can absorb water and electrolytes when administered with glucose, even during severe secretory diarrhea.

The optimal composition of rehydration fluid for gastrointestinal losses is a sodium concentration between 50 and 90 mEq/L. The lower concentration may be more palatable, but the higher concentration is most effective with moderate dehydration. Maximal glucose concentration is 2 to 2.5%. Higher concentrations may have an osmotic effect, making diarrhea worse. Cereal-based ORS contains complex carbohydrate molecules from rice or grains that do not create an excessive osmotic load, but are digested as simple glucose. At least 20 mEq/L of potassium is necessary and 30 mEq/L of bicarbonate is optimal.

The World Health Organization (WHO) has developed electrolyte salts specifically for diarrheal illness that contain 90 mEq of sodium, 20 mEq of potassium, 80 mEq of chloride, 30 mEq of bicarbonate or trisodium citrate, and 111 mmol (2%) of glucose, which must be mixed with one liter (approximately one quart) of disinfected water. Packets of these oral rehydration salts are distributed throughout the world by WHO and UNICEF, commonly under the name Oralyte. More expensive premixed solutions are available but are not practical for wilderness or foreign travel. Sports drinks and other "clear liquids" contain insufficient sodium and potassium and excessive glucose for treatment of diarrheal induced dehydration, but they are better than plain water.

If premeasured salts are not available, a substitute recommended by the Centers for Disease Control and Prevention (CDC) consists of alternating glasses of the following two fluids:

Glass #1:   8 oz fruit juice (such as apple, orange, or lemon)
½ tsp honey or corn syrup
1 pinch salt

Glass #2:   8 oz water (boiled or treated)
¼ tsp baking soda

However, these ingredients may not be available to remote travelers.

Plain salt and sugar solutions, similar to those used for heat/exercise replacement, can be used for mild dehydration but are not adequate for serious dehydration or replacement of continuing high losses. Where nothing else is available, rice water, fruit juice, colas, or coconut milk may have to suffice for supplementation in cases of mild dehydration or partial maintenance.

II. GUIDELINES FOR FLUID REPLACEMENT

Achieve replacement of estimated fluid deficit in about four hours by giving 50 ml/kg (1.6 oz/.2.2 lb) body weight for mild dehydration and 100 ml/kg (3.2 oz/2.2 lb) for moderate dehydration. This means that for mild dehydration, an adult should drink 250 ml (approximately one-half pint) of oral rehydration solution every thirty minutes for the first four to six hours. Children should drink 200 to 250 ml (one-third to one-half pint)/hour. In addition, they may drink water as desired. Give infants under three months a 100 ml (approximately 4 oz) dose each hour with every third dose replaced by plain water. Ingestion of frequent, small amounts, rather than rapid ingestion of a large volume, minimizes vomiting. Fluid deficit is replaced within twelve hours in 90 percent of patients. Determine maintenance fluids by estimating or measuring stool losses plus normal maintenance requirements. Since this is not often possible in the field, give 10 to 15 ml/kg (0.32 to .48 oz/2.2 lb) body weight/diarrheal stool.

At least 90 percent of patients during diarrhea epidemics can be successfully rehydrated using only ORS. Failure of ORS occurs when stool losses exceed oral intake. Vomiting, unless frequent and protracted, does not preclude rehydration with oral solutions. Fluids may be administered by nasogastric tube when the patient is unable or unwilling to drink adequate fluids. Intravenous fluids can be reserved for the initial hydration of patients with shock, obtundation, seizures, or intractable vomiting. When IV fluids are necessary, ORS usually can be initiated within four hours and exclusively used within twenty-four hours.

III. CONTROVERSIES

A. Does ORS cause hypernatremia in patients without cholera? Many physicians in developed countries avoid ORS because of an unsubstantiated concern for hypernatremia in small children. This concern has led to lower sodium concentrations (50 to 75 mEq/L) in commercial ORS sold in the United States and recommendations to use the higher concentration only for initial rehydration then lower concentrations for maintenance. This complexity can be avoided if plain water or formula is alternated with ORS in the maintenance phase of treatment.

B. Are electrolyte replacement drinks necessary for wilderness activities? Cases of severe hyponatremia in endurance athletes and recreational hikers in hot climates have been reported and were probably caused by "water intoxication." As sweat losses increase with environmental heat stress and prolonged exercise, electrolyte replacement becomes more important. Most wilderness sports such as hiking, climbing, or skiing offer frequent opportunities to rest and ingest food and fluids. If snack foods are eaten regularly, plain water will be safe for fluid replacement. Unfortunately, many hikers favor snack foods that are high in carbohydrates and fats (such as candy) but low in sodium. Some individuals, noting the edema present in their hands and feet associated with heat or altitude exposure, attempt to restrict their sodium intake. The development of heat exhaustion causes nausea, preventing food intake. If frequent snack and meal breaks are not planned, recommend electrolyte replacement fluids for sustained wilderness activities in hot climates.

Chapter 17

BOTANICAL ENCOUNTERS

I. GENERAL INFORMATION

A few plant families cause trouble. The majority of problems are due to contact but some are due to ingestion, mostly of fungi. Treatment in the field depends on the nature and severity of the problem. Many contact episodes can be treated on the spot. Virtually all contacts by ingestion require immediate evacuation.

II. PLANT-INDUCED DERMATITIS

Most injuries result from simple mechanical or chemical trauma, sensitization to allergens or a photochemical response. Dermal reactions may be immunologic, nonimmunologic, or both. Injuries may be further complicated by secondary infections, that is, reactions and further damage by excoriation or improper treatment. Identification of the offending plant is important both for treatment and future avoidance.

A. Mechanical Injury and Treatment

Many plants possess spines, thorns, bristles, barbs, or sharp edges. Contact can cause punctures or lacerations that often contain embedded plant material. Other plants contain specialized structures to deliver irritants that cause both mechanical and chemical injury. Numerous spines, thorns, and fine hairs (called glochids) in the cactus genus *Opuntia* can cause aseptic granulomatous lesions resembling scabies.

Follow basic wound care principles when treating punctures and lacerations. Clean all wounds and remove any foreign material. Apply, then carefully remove, tape to extract fine foreign bodies. Deeply embedded material must be excised to avoid serious complications such as osteoblastic and osteolytic changes in bone, synovitis in joints and localized or generalized infections. If removal is not possible in a remote location, the victim must be transported for definitive care. Provide pain control as necessary and if definitive care cannot be reached within two to three days, initiate antibiotic prophylaxis as soon as possible to reduce the chance of infection. Most infections will be caused by dermatologic organisms and are usually well covered by first generation cephalosporins. Augmented pencillins, fluoroquinolones, and macrolide antibiotics are alternatives.

If the foreign body can be removed, antibiotic treatment should be reserved for secondary infections. Tetanus prophylaxis is required for these injuries.

Many plants contain irritants that cause reactions through their chemical or physical properties. For example, members of the family Araceae (e.g., *Dieffenbachia* or dumbcane) possess bundles of needle-like calcium oxalate crystals in their cells (raphides) that cause intense pain and itching due to their microinvasive properties. Often children learn this through an unfortunate tasting experiment. These substances affect most people and are not dependent upon an individual being "allergic" to the offending agent. The reaction generally happens within seconds to minutes of the exposure, compared to "allergic" reactions that usually develop twenty to thirty minutes after contact. The two cannot be differentiated by inspection alone. Treatment consists of general cleaning with cool compresses for comfort and analgesics as necessary. Most reactions are self-limited but can be quite painful for twelve to twenty-four hours. Intense itching can be relieved with antihistamines.

Contaminated eyes should be copiously irrigated. A cycloplegic such as scopolamine 0.25% drops (see Wilderness Eye Injuries, Chapter 9) may greatly relieve pain along with the use of artificial tears. Patching is not helpful unless a foreign body cannot be removed.

B. Chemical Injury and Treatment

Allergic dermatitis: This phenomenon occurs after previous sensitization to an allergen. These agents are usually in the form of a hapten that combines with skin proteins to form an antigen. This is a cellular (type IV) reaction mediated by T-lymphocytes. In those individuals who tend to be atopic, the reaction can be eczematous.

In the United States the family Anacardiaceae containing poison ivy *(Toxicodendron radicans)* and poison oak *(T. diversilobum)* causes more dermatitis more than any other plant, household, or industrial chemicals. The offending agents here are various catechols. The severity of reaction to this family depends on the size and thickness of the cornified skin exposed, and the dose of toxin received. Following contact a cutaneous response occurs in twelve to twenty-four hours. This latent period can be helpful in determining the mechanism of reaction. Initially an area of erythema develops usually with some edema.

During the next twenty-four hours vesicles or bullae develop containing a nonallergic serous fluid that does not spread the dermatitis, contrary to popular belief. Exudation may be marked and itching is intense. After several days crusting develops and resolution occurs in ten to fourteen days barring complications. Previously affected sites distant from the currently affected area may flare as well.

Cutaneous penetration takes about ten minutes. Therefore if exposure is immediately recognized prompt washing may reduce the severity or prevent a reaction. Washing with water is recommended, but avoid soaps as they remove protective oils from the skin. Apply organic solvents such as alcohol carefully to avoid spreading the agent. Both topical and oral steroids are maximally effective during this period. Generally "dose-packs" are inadequate in both dose and duration except in mild cases. Prednisone should be started with an oral dose of 0.75–1 mg/kg/day (usually 60 to 80 mg) for ten days and then tapered by 10 mg every other day to prevent recurrence.

Avoidance of the plant is the best policy, and it is recommended that you discard any objects or clothing that came into contact with the material.

Numerous other plants can also cause reactions. It is vital to remember that some individuals may have an anaphylactic reaction to a dermal exposure. Should this occur, the first-line treatment is epinephrine (1:1000) 0.2–0.5 ml SQ or IM.

Contact Urticaria: This reaction may be immunologic or nonimmunologic. It is characterized by a central irregular raised wheal that is mildly blanched, surrounded by an irregular, more erythematous flare. The process is caused by the release of histamines and other vasoactive agents. The reaction produces a sensation ranging from mildly itchy to intensely painful such as those reactions caused by the Urticaceae (nettle) family. Occasionally an ipsilateral self-limiting lymphadenopathy can develop. Generally, a good cleansing of the area is all that is necessary as this process is self-limited. Administer pain and itch medication.

Photodermatitis: Some plant species contain psoralens that sensitize the skin to ultraviolet light. This is a phototoxic reaction, facilitated by moisture, when these substances come in contact with the skin. With sun exposure, mild to severe burns can occur. Areas exposed need to be protected from the sun for approximately two weeks.

Treatment is the same as for any sunburn. Cool compresses and administration of nonsteroidal anti-inflammatories such as ibuprofen or aspirin can be helpful.

III. PLANT INGESTIONS

Between 1994 and 1999 one million people in the United States ingested potentially dangerous plants: Only twenty-seven died, and major morbidity was rare. While the majority of ingested toxins were from fungi (mushrooms), numerous deadly toxins exist, such as ricin and abrin from *Ricinus* and *Abru,* cicutoxin from *Cicuta douglasii* (water hemlock), gyratoxins from the Rhododendron family, aconitine from the genus *Acontium* (wolfsbane and monkshood) and numerous alkaloids that all tend to present with GI symptoms. Toxicity is low with inadvertent exposures but can be fatal after a large dose as often happens with a case of mistaken identity, "folk" remedies, and ritualistic ingestions. Later, more serious symptoms can develop with deadly consequences.

Diagnosis

A presumptive diagnosis can be made based upon the history and early presenting signs and symptoms. To plan treatment, every effort should be made to note the overall shape of the tree or shrub and collect any available flowers, fruits, and foliage. Several highly toxic or fatal species look almost identical to other harmless and even delicious plants. Toxicities within and among species can vary greatly depending upon location, and a poor correlation exists between taxonomy and toxicity. Consequently clinical judgment and re-evaluation of the victim are of the utmost importance.

Mushroom Ingestions

If mushroom poisoning is suspected, urgently evacuate to definitive medical care. Initiate seizure precautions. Vomiting is a common result of mushroom poisoning. A late onset of gastric cramping and vomiting may be a more serious prognostic indicator than early onset of symptoms. Almost *none* of the mushroom toxins are changed by heat or drying. Therefore, cooking the plants does not remove the danger, and toxicity can occur from inhalation of mushroom fumes as well as from ingestion.

Treatment

Treatment in the field is, of necessity, limited because the diagnosis may be uncertain and the appropriate therapeutic agents—such as activated charcoal—are rarely, if ever, included in a first-aid kit (for the use of ipecac see below).

If vomiting can be induced within the first few minutes after ingestion, in an alert patient, some benefit may be achieved. The induction of vomiting after thirty minutes is of no benefit.

All victims of known or suspected toxic ingestion should be evacuated as rapidly as possible. If the victim develops seizures, benzodiazepines may be helpful for their control. An unconscious patient must be checked frequently to maintain and protect the airway, which may become compromised by excessive salivation or secretions.

IV. CONTROVERSIES

Is vomiting a beneficial reflex? Should syrup of ipecac be administered in the treatment of poisoning? A position statement by the American Academy of Clinical Toxicology and the European Association of Poisons Centres and Clinical Toxicologists (1997) indicates that there was insufficient data to support or exclude ipecac administration soon after poison ingestion. Its use may delay the administration or reduce the effectiveness of activated charcoal. The above position statement advises against the routine use of syrup of ipecac in the management of poisoned patients. It is unclear whether naturally occurring vomiting or induced vomiting is beneficial in a wilderness setting.

Chapter 18

WILD LAND ANIMAL ATTACKS

I. GENERAL INFORMATION

Although few truly large and wild animals remain in the contiguous United States, injuries from attacks by alligators, bison, bears, and cougars (mountain lions) occur annually. In Alaska and overseas, wild animal attacks are a more significant cause of morbidity and mortality. Many of these involve predation by the big cats or by bears, but other species such as elephant, rhinoceros, wild pig, or hippopotamus also attack humans.

Injuries from large wild animal attack result from a variety of mechanisms including biting, clawing, chewing, goring, tossing, or trampling. As a result the victim often sustains major trauma far beyond a simple bite, involving multiple organ systems and locations. Wounds are always contaminated with oral or soil pathogens.

Rabies should be considered a possibility when the bite is sustained from a small mammal (see below).

A. Wild Cats

Wild cats spring from behind to attack the neck of their prey, sharply hyperextending the neck to fracture the cervical spine and transect the spinal cord and great vessels with their teeth.

B. Horned Animals

Goring injuries from animals such as bull, American buffalo, bison, elephant, or rhinoceros produce deep puncture wounds. These may rip along fascial planes or penetrate deeply, and evisceration is common. Trampling or tossing by these animals also results in blunt trauma to the victim.

C. Bears

Bears of all types claw, bite, crush, and tear their victims. Attacks are often aimed preferentially at the head, with extensive facial injuries and scalping. Chewing on extremities is also described.

II. PREVENTION

For all wild animal attacks, prevention can be summarized: Don't get too close; stay out of the way. Approaching too closely while photographing is particularly risky. Alertness and awareness of the animal habitat during wilderness travel will prevent many encounters. Reduce unexpected animal encounters on the trail by avoiding large animal paths and areas dotted with fresh scat. Avoid attracting animals by keeping campsites clean and by hanging all food and aromatic substances well above the ground and away from tents. Traveling in groups is safer than traveling alone.

General recommendations in case of a nonpredatory attack or encounter include attempting to remove the perceived threat to the animal, i.e., you. In an unanticipated encounter, slowly and quietly back away. Running away will often elicit a predatory response. "Playing dead" by dropping to the ground, rolling into a knee-to-chest ball, and covering your head and face with your arms is advised in a sudden grizzly encounter. These maneuvers all "remove the threat."

If an attack is unprovoked, with humans seen as prey, aggressively fighting back is recommended. Behavior such as advancing rather than fleeing, making loud noises, or waving arms to appear larger and more threatening may forestall an attack. Vigorous resistance with physical fighting, including striking the attacking animal with fists or any object or weapon, has been effective in repelling attacks by cougars, lions, tigers, brown and black bears, and even crocodiles. Cayenne pepper spray may be useful if approached by a bear. Many people carry firearms in "bear country." Both pepper spray and firearms may provide a false sense of security. Both must be used correctly by persons trained in their use to be effective.

Avoidance is best. Common sense dictates care in traveling, camping, food storage, cooking, and sleeping. Preparation with a plan of action in case of an attack is strongly advised. Be familiar with the type of animals you are likely to encounter and the best methods of handling an encounter if it occurs.

III. GUIDELINES FOR ASSESSMENT AND TREATMENT

Scene safety is an initial consideration for rescuers: Is the animal gone or liable to attack again? Do not spend time tracking the attacking animal unless adequate assistance to the victim is simultaneously available and rescuers are experienced and competent in such activity.

Attend to ABCs as always. Airway management may be complicated with head, facial, neck, or chest injuries. Assume all victims of large wild animal attacks have sustained multiple traumas. Beyond the obvious bite, claw, or goring wounds, the victim needs assessment for fractures, neurovascular damage, and internal head, chest, and abdominal injury. Try to determine the mechanisms of injury. Soft tissue damage far beyond the obvious may result from trampling, butting, or tossing with ground impact. Bites regularly penetrate more deeply than apparent. Recognize the factor of psychological trauma, even in the field.

Wound cleaning is the single most important step in preventing infection: its importance cannot be overemphasized (see Wilderness Wound Management, Chapter 6). Splint large open wounds and fractures (see Orthopedic Injuries, Chapter 8). Cover abdominal eviscerations and eye injuries with a moist, clean dressing—and evacuate rapidly.

Vigorously irrigate animal bites with water safe to drink, then scrub with soap and water, followed by a sixty- to ninety-second rinse with a 1% concentration of povidone-iodine or .5% chlorhexidine gluconate, if available. Except where necessary to control hemorrhage or to allow extrication, never close or tightly approximate an animal bite wound. Devitalized, necrotic tissue from bite and crush injuries is common, requiring debridement. These injuries are all contaminated. Give amoxicillin-clavulanate, a second or third generation cephalosporin, a quinolone, a penicillinase resistant penicillin, or a tetracycline antibiotic (erythromycin is not an acceptable alternative). All wild cats, from cougars in the United States and Canada, to leopards, lions, and tigers in Africa and Asia, inflict bite wounds contaminated with *Pasteurella multocida*. Parenteral antibiotic treatment is indicated with penicillin, or if penicillin allergic, a cephalosporin. Update tetanus prior to travel as these injuries are high-risk wounds for tetanus.

IV. RABIES

Consider rabies in bites in pets (dogs, cats, ferrets) if: 1) the attack was unprovoked (a bite is considered provoked if there was any attempt to feed, pet, run by, or capture the animal); or 2) the animal was acting unnaturally prior to the bite. Consider all other animals inflicting bites, with the exception of rodents and lagomorphs (rabbits), rabid unless they can be caught and tested for rabies. Ship the heads to a public health lab. Observation in quarantine for other animals, including wolf hybrids, is not reliable. Telephone local public health services for advice after a rodent bite. In case of a suspicious bite, administer rabies immune globulin as soon as possible and certainly within seventy-two hours and simultaneously with rabies vaccine in nonimmunized people. The CDC recommends rabies prophylaxis for all carnivore bites. *Aggressive and immediate wound cleaning will reduce the chance of contracting rabies.* Consider rabies prophylaxis prior to travel in remote regions where rabies is prevalent. Current CDC recommendations are available from the Division of Viral and Rickettsial Diseases at (404) 639–1050 during regular business hours or (404) 639–2888 nights, weekends, and holidays. This information is also on the CDC Web site at www.cdc.gov/ncidod/dvrd/rabies.

V. GUIDELINES FOR EVACUATION

Victims of large wild animal attack, even with stable vital signs, usually require urgent evacuation from the field for surgical wound treatment, as well as multiple trauma evaluation. Lesser wounds or bites may require evacuation for antibiotic treatment, rabies prophylaxis, cosmetic closure, or wound exploration and cleaning.

If rescue and evacuation will require days, close observation of vital signs, daily wound care with additional field irrigation, cleaning, debridement, dressing changes as needed, and antibiotic administration are advised.

Chapter 19

MARINE ENVENOMATIONS AND POISONINGS

I. GENERAL INFORMATION

Marine creatures may cause illness both by injection (envenomation) and ingestion (poisoning) of the multitude of toxins they elaborate. There is a broad range of species involved and these are widely distributed. In general, tropical and subtropical environments are the highest risk areas. Many of the venoms and toxins involved are still poorly characterized, yet they're recognizable themes across species in patterns of envenomation and management.

II. GUIDELINES FOR PREVENTION

Prevention of marine envenomations and poisonings requires local knowledge. In general, common sense is required. Few marine creatures are aggressive unless disturbed. Stout footwear is an obvious precaution when walking through shallows, especially coral or rocks. Do not handle marine creatures—observe them from a distance. During high risk periods wear "stinger suits" to minimize the risk of jellyfish envenomation and where possible swim at safe beaches or in protected enclosures. Know which species of fish and seafood can be safely eaten at any given time. Perhaps most importantly, know the risks of your local environment. Know the appropriate first aid and be aware of the definitive care of each condition.

III. GUIDELINES FOR ASSESSMENT AND TREATMENT

Other than attention to the ABCs, care of the victim of a marine envenomation or poisoning may include: prevention of further envenomation, venom neutralization, pain relief, specific antivenoms, specific adjunctive drug therapy, and surgical wound care.

A. Jellyfish

This group covers an enormous range of genus and species. They share a common means of envenomation through thousands of tiny stinging capsules (nematocysts), which come into contact with exposed flesh that passes through their trailing tentacles. Some of the medically more important include the box jellyfish (Chironex), man-o-war, and the irukandji. Immediate and often severe local pain is the rule with jellyfish stings. Most jellyfish will also cause a prominent skin rash. The most severe envenomations (especially those of the box jellyfish) may lead to respiratory failure and cardiovascular collapse.

For all types of box jellyfish stings, vinegar (4 to 6% acetic acid) splashed liberally over the areas where stingers are adherent reliably inhibits nematocyst discharge and inactivates remaining undischarged nematocysts. This therapy is not proven to be effective or harmful in other jellyfish envenomations. Once inactivated, remaining stingers should be plucked off with gloved fingers or forceps. Dried nematocysts may be reactivated by water exposure so stingers should be physically removed and not washed off. Pressure immobilization bandaging as used in Elapid snakebites may be useful first aid, especially in box jellyfish envenomation.

B. Venomous Fish Stings

Many fish and rays possess sharp stinging spines capable of causing local trauma and, through injection of venom, intense local pain. Deaths have been associated with many species either due to direct local trauma or to the effects of envenomation. Secondary local infection and local tissue damage is often described. Retained local foreign bodies are common.

Pain relief in these cases is usually obtained by immersion of the affected area in hot water. Whether this technique works by venom neutralization or other local effects is uncertain. Care must be taken to test the hot water beforehand. The water should be as hot as can be comfortably tolerated (40 to 43°C, 104 to 110°F), but not so hot as to cause burns, particularly if the area is anaesthetized. Narcotic analgesia or injected local anesthesia may be required to ensure pain control. Antivenom, which is injected IM, is available and is effective against stone fish. Any venomous fish sting requires careful wound examination and even surgical care to ensure retained foreign bodies are avoided.

C. Sea Snakes

Bites from these creatures are a common cause of envenomation on a worldwide scale, especially in the Indo-Pacific regions. Sea snakes are generally nonaggressive and will only attack if provoked or interfered with. The effects of their venom, clinical manifestations, and treatment are the same as for other Elapid snakes (see Reptile Envenomations, Chapter 20). In particular, pressure immobilization bandaging and rapid transfer to a medical facility for specific antivenom therapy may be lifesaving.

D. Mollusk Envenomations

The two most notable are coneshells and blue ring octopus, both of which may inject rapid acting neurotoxins. These produce a progressive paralysis that has been associated with a number of deaths. The key to management is recognition and support of ventilation (using mouth to mouth in the field if required). Pressure immobilization bandaging may help to limit venom spread and the onset of toxic effects (see Reptile Envenomations, Chapter 20).

E. Marine Poison Ingestions

On a worldwide scale these are likely to be the single largest cause of mortality associated with encounters with marine creatures. Poisoning with tetrodotoxin occurs from eating the flesh of incorrectly prepared pufferfish ("fugu"). Although slower in onset, the manifestations and required management will be similar to that seen with blue ring octopus envenomation. Again the key lifesaving intervention is artificial support of ventilation.

Paralytic shellfish poisoning is due to ingestion of mollusks that have themselves ingested and concentrated the poison saxitoxin that is produced by microscopic dinoflagellates. This toxin produces a rapid onset of paralysis that is managed in the same way as pufferfish poisoning (see above).

Cigautera poisoning occurs from eating fish that have concentrated toxins passed up the food chain from dinoflagellates. The illness is particularly common in parts of the South Pacific and West Indies. Specific species of fish are recognized as the common causes in specific geographic locations with the onset being one to twenty-four hours after the fish ingestion. Symptoms vary but commonly include: diarrhea, nausea, abdominal pain, muscle aches, numbness or burning of the skin, irritability, and loss of balance. Reversal of heat and cold sensation can develop. The gastrointestinal symptoms usually only last a day or two while the neurological symptoms may persist for weeks. Drinking alcohol will worsen symptoms. The best treatment is prevention by avoiding eating fish that are likely to be affected.

Chapter 20

REPTILE ENVENOMATIONS

I. GENERAL INFORMATION

There are approximately 300,000 human snakebites worldwide each year from 2,700 known species. In the United States it is estimated that there are 45,000 bites of humans with 8,000 envenomations and five to twelve deaths per year. The incidence of bites and fatality rates is much higher in other parts of the world. In general, fatalities are more frequent where the snakes are more venomous, or where lay knowledge regarding venomous bites and access to medical care are lacking. Venomous snakes can be broadly divided into Crotalidae (pit vipers—including rattlesnakes, cottonmouths, and copperheads) and the family Elapidae (which includes coral snakes and all venomous Australian snakes). There are about 3,000 known species of lizards, but only members of the family Helodermatidae (including Gila monsters) are considered venomous. They are found exclusively in the southwestern United States and Mexico. No human fatalities have been reported. Fatalities from U.S. crotalid envenomation are not common, but complications may be severe.

A. Pit Vipers

Crotalids have a triangular head, cat-like vertical pupils, hinged fangs, and a heat-sensitive "pit" on each side of the head between the tip of the nose and the eye. Rattlesnakes have a variable number of rattles depending upon age and number of molts. They sometimes strike without rattling. About 60 percent of this country's venomous bites are attributed to rattlesnakes. Cottonmouths (water moccasins) and copperheads are the other two commonly encountered North American pit vipers. Copperhead and cottonmouth venoms are quite similar and weaker than most rattlesnake venoms. Bites by cottonmouths tend to be more serious than copperhead bites because the cottonmouth is a bigger snake.

B. Elapidae

These species are widely distributed, most particularly in the Southern

Hemisphere. They are notable for bites that cause profound systemic effects such as neuromuscular paralysis and coagulopathy and myonecrosis, but often with minimal local effects. Identification of species even by trained observers is notoriously difficult and is not to be used to guide therapy. The several species of coral snakes are brightly colored, with black noses and alternating red-yellow-red-black bands around their bodies (remember "red on yellow can kill a fellow"). They have relatively small mouths with fixed fangs. From southern Mexico through tropical South America the rules for distinguishing coral snakes are highly unreliable. Unless you are a knowledgeable herpetologist, it is best not to pick up colorful snakes in tropical America.

C. Gila Monsters

These lizards are not large, seldom reaching twenty inches in length. They have blunt heads, beady eyes, and powerful digging claws on short legs. They are shy and appear sluggish but are capable of swift, determined lunges when threatened or handled.

II. PREVENTION

Wilderness travelers are rarely bitten by venomous reptiles. Avoid reptile bites by: 1) staying away from infested areas; 2) not hiking during times of peak reptile activity (usually at night); 3) watching clearly where one steps; 4) never reaching into concealed areas (gathering firewood at night, for example); 5) checking bedding, clothing, and footwear before use; and 6) never handling a venomous reptile, even if it is presumed dead (reflex allows some pit vipers to strike even after death). The chance of envenomation from a strike can be minimized by wearing high leather boots and long pants. Envenomation is more apt to occur in persons who are intoxicated and in young children. It is helpful to know the distribution, markings, and characteristics of venomous reptiles in intended areas of wilderness travel.

III. GUIDELINES FOR ASSESSMENT AND TREATMENT

A. Pit Vipers

As many as 20 to 30 percent of crotalid bites cause no envenomation. Most, but not all, crotalid envenomations result in immediate pain at the bite site, and a rapid onset (within ten to fifteen minutes) of swelling and ecchymosis. Rarely, signs of envenomation are delayed for several hours. Typical paired fang wounds are not always present. A single puncture or a scratch may be the only mark, and the degree of envenomation does not correlate with the size, quality, and number of fang marks.

Assessment of envenomation by a pit viper is the first step in managing a bite in the field. Mark the advancing border of edema and sequentially measure and mark the circumference at the site and at least one location above the bite to detect spreading edema. Reassess these measurements every fifteen minutes. Gently cleanse the area. Apply a sterile or clean dressing. The basic tenet is to provide calm, rapid transport to a medical facility. For an extremity bite, splint the limb. Do not use pressure dressings, tourniquets, applications of cold, electric shocks, or incisions of the bite site, as these techniques have no known efficacy. Lymphatic constricting bands (barely indenting the skin) are advocated by some, although their use has not been proven to have any definite advantage in pit viper envenomations. The only scientifically proven method for extracting venom from a bite site is with the Extractor device (Sawyer Products). In animal studies, it has been demonstrated that up to 30 percent of total injected venom can be removed if the device is used within three minutes after the bite occurs.

Encourage the patient to rest and stay calm. Keep the extremity at heart level or lower. Severe manifestations of poisoning may not occur for several hours, so obtaining treatment at a hospital is a priority. If evacuation requires the patient to walk out, proceed immediately.

For those with the skill and equipment start one large-bore (16 g or larger) IV in an unaffected limb. Start at least two large-bore IVs in a patient presenting with shock. Administer either normal saline or Ringer's lactate solution (LR) to support systolic blood pressure above 90 mm Hg. Intubation or vasopressors are rarely necessary in crotalid envenomations. Field use of intravenous antivenin is not recommended.

B. Elapidae

Immediate local symptoms and signs from these bites may be minimal. The degree and rapidity of the onset of systemic symptoms will vary according to the species, bite site, and effectiveness of the bite. Systemic symptoms such as nausea, vomiting, sweating, myalgias, and general malaise are common. Signs of paralysis such as generalized weakness, blurred vision, and respiratory difficulties may become obvious. There may be no signs of overwhelming coagulopathy until a catastrophe such as an intracerebral bleed occurs. In all cases of suspected bite assume envenomation and treat accordingly. There is strong evidence that in elapid bites appropriate first aid may be lifesaving. An elastic bandage applied at a similar tension to that for a sprained ankle should commence at the bite site and extend along the length of the limb and back again to the bite. Splint the limb and keep the patient still. The patient must not self-evacuate under any circumstances as activity will enhance movement of the venom centrally. With well-conducted first aid, venom will be trapped and broken down locally and the risk of life threatening envenomation will be minimized. With the acknowledged problems in elapid species identification and of antivenin storage, the field use of antivenin is not recommended.

C. Gila Monsters

Gila monsters have no injection mechanism for their venom, but they have very powerful jaws and they chew and tear at their victims, drooling venom and producing a substantial amount of pain. Envenomation produces pain, swelling, vomiting, increased heart rate, vertigo, shortness of breath, and loss of consciousness. Follow the recommendations for pit viper envenomation. Fatal Gila monster encounters are extremely rare.

Chapter 21

ARTHROPOD ENVENOMATIONS

I. GENERAL INFORMATION

In the United States, arthropods (invertebrates with jointed legs and segmented bodies) cause more deaths by envenomation than reptiles. Hymenoptera (bees, wasps, etc.), the Arachnida (spiders and scorpions), and Chilopoda (centipedes) cause the most significant envenomations.

Neither *Latrodectus* (North American black widow, Australian redback, New Zealand kati, South African knoppie) nor *Loxosceles* (brown recluse) are aggressive toward humans. These spiders live in crevices under ground cover, trash piles, barns, porches, and outside toilets. Prevention includes inspection, clearing, and care, especially around these areas. Nearly half of all bites could be prevented if toilets and clothing were inspected prior to use.

II. GUIDELINES FOR ASSESSMENT AND TREATMENT

A. Stinging Insects

The most common insect stings are from the Hymenoptera. Although it takes about 300 to 500 stings to make a lethal dose of the complex venom, hypersensitivity, which occurs in approximately 1 percent of the general public, may result in a life-threatening anaphylactic reaction from a solitary sting. This is more common in adults than in children.

The Hymenoptera comprise four families: 1) honeybees, which account for the most stings and leave the stinger attached to their victims; 2) bumblebees; 3) hornets, yellow jackets, and wasps; and 4) fire ants, whose alkaloid venom results in a sterile, burning, vesicular lesion.

Nearly all Hymenoptera stings result in local pain, swelling, and redness. The honeybee stinger should be removed as soon as possible by the most expedient means to prevent the injection of still more venom. The site may be treated locally with gentle cleansing, application of cold, elevation, and immobilization. Calm the patient. Common remedies, such as applying a slurry of baking soda or meat tenderizer, often reduce pain.

Commercial "sting sticks" containing a topical anesthetic like xylocaine may be used unless the patient is known to be allergic to the drug. Oral aspirin or ibuprofen usually help control pain. The use of a noninvasive suction cup, the Sawyer Extractor, helps alleviate pain and is effective in removing a portion of the venom if applied within three minutes.

Patients with serious allergic reactions have pruritis, hives, angioedema, and respiratory distress. For these individuals apply a light constrictive band (not a tourniquet) proximal to the site. Oral antihistamines (such as diphenhydramine) may be helpful. If the patient is carrying injectable epinephrine, administer it if angioedema, respiratory distress, or hypotension develops. Arrange for evacuation as soon as possible. Maintaining ABCs may be extremely difficult without advanced knowledge and equipment.

If any signs of anaphylactic reaction are identified, rescuers carrying epinephrine should administer the drug IM (0.3 to 0.5 mg for an adult, 0.01 mg/kg up to the adult maximum for a child) or via preloaded syringes as often as necessary, depending on the patient's status.

B. Spider Bites

There are approximately 100,000 species of spiders worldwide, with a density of up to two million spiders per acre in some areas. In the United States, the most significant venomous spiders are the black widow (*Latrodectus mactans*) and the fiddleback, or brown recluse (*Loxosceles reclusa*). The venoms of these spiders are potent toxins with numerous antigenic components capable of causing either a systemic manifestation or a local venom reaction.

Black widow is itself a misnomer because only three of the five species of widow spider (Family Therdiidae) are actually black, the others being brown and gray. The female spider is the larger of the sexes, often measuring 1 to 1.5 cm (one-third to one-half inch) long, with a leg span of 4 to 5 cm (1.5 to 2 inches). The female has a unique hourglass mark, usually red, on the ventral abdominal surface. Newly-hatched spiders are almost entirely red, darkening with progressive molts. Males are 3 to 5 mm ($\frac{1}{10}$ to $\frac{2}{10}$ inches) long with white stripes along the lateral aspect of the abdomen.

Only adult females can envenomate. The bite usually feels like a mild pinprick (and may not be noticed) with subsequent slight redness that usually disappears within a few minutes to an hour. Systemic symptoms of envenomation begin ten to sixty minutes after the bite of the female and are caused by the release of the neurotransmitters acetylcholine and norepinephrine. A few minutes after the bite a small weal appears, followed within fifteen to sixty minutes by a band of excruciating cramping pain that remains localized or spreads to involve the thigh, shoulder, back, and abdominal muscles. A board-like abdomen often simulates an acute abdomen. Bites on the arm can produce chest pain that mimics a myocardial infarction. Hypertension, respiratory distress, seizures, and, occasionally in the very young or old, cardiopulmonary arrest are all possible complications. These symptoms frequently subside in twenty-four hours, but in a few cases recur for several days to months. The very young, very old, and those with hypertension have the greatest risk of morbidity from *Latrodectus* envenomation.

Reassure the patient and have him or her rest as much as possible. Assess ABCs and monitor vital signs. Attempt to assess whether the individual was indeed bitten by a spider or whether another process is occurring. Cold applied to the bite site may reduce localized pain somewhat. If significant pain is present, immobilize the involved extremity. Oral analgesics are useful for muscle pain.

If available, narcotics may be necessary for pain control, but care must be taken to avoid hypotension and respiratory depression. A number of therapies for *Latrodectus* envenomation (such as muscle relaxants and IV calcium gluconate) have been tried with limited success. There is little doubt that antivenin is the most effective therapy; however, the safety of the IV antivenin used in North America is of concern. In Australasia and Japan, a different antivenin is used IM with an excellent safety and efficacy record. Due to the difficulties of storing antivenin, its field use cannot be recommended. Immediate evacuation is recommended for signs of serious envenomation.

Fiddlebacks are often called brown recluses, but these spiders are not always distinctively brown. They may have a distinctive violin or fiddle-shaped mark on the dorsal cephalothorax. They average 12 mm (one-half inch) long with a leg span of up to 5 cm (two inches). The bite of both sexes is equally venomous, although usually painless. Within a few hours, a macule or vesicle may appear at the site. In a severe bite, erythema and blistering follow within six to twelve hours. The classic picture is a hemorrhagic vesicle surrounded by a white or pale ischemic zone, and then by an erythematous region—the so-called bull's-eye lesion. By inspection of the lesion alone, however, it is usually impossible to differentiate a *Loxosceles* bite from many other skin lesions and bites. Pruritus and rash can also occur. Nausea, vomiting, headache, and fever are common systemic symptoms. The lesion either resolves or becomes necrotic and indurated. This may require excision or grafting. Symptoms of envenomation with fiddleback bites are caused by cell and tissue injury and direct lytic action of sphingomyelinase on red cell membranes. Rarely, and mostly in children, massive intravascular hemolysis develops after necrosis of the local bite. Deaths have been reported in the United States.

Treatment consists of local wound care. If the wound becomes necrotic and extends to more than 1 cm (one-third inch) in diameter, the use of oral dapsone may be indicated. Do not use dapsone unless the person has been tested for Glucose-6 Phosphatase deficiency. The short-term application of ice packs to the bite site is as effective as any other form of therapy. The patient may be placed on a corticosteroid, such as prednisone 1 mg/kg daily for five days, during the acute phase.

C. Scorpion Stings

Approximately 650 species of scorpions inhabit the world, mainly distributed in tropical and subtropical areas. An estimated forty of these species live in the United States, distributed across 75 percent of the country but concentrated in the warmer regions. All scorpions inject venom through a single sharp stinger at the tip of the "tail," which is actually an extension of the abdomen. Contact with scorpions is usually accidental. They feed at night. During the daytime they may take shelter in clothing, boots, and bedding. Outdoors, they may often be found under rocks and logs. Checking their hiding places in known scorpion areas is good advice for any traveler. Although the sting is painful, few species inject sufficient venom to be of concern to humans. The only potentially lethal U.S. scorpion is *Centruroides exilicauda* (or *sculpturatus*). *C. gertschi* is generally considered a variety of *sculpturatus*. This scorpion is found primarily in Arizona. It is most active May through August, hibernating in winter. Since specific identification is difficult, the traveler is advised to inquire locally about what dangerous species are present before traveling into scorpion territory. As with black widow spiders, most deaths and serious reactions from *Centruroides* stings are in small children, the elderly, and hypertensives.

Any sting typically produces a burning pain, minimal swelling, redness, vesicles, numbness, tingling, and, uncommonly, weakness or numbness of the affected extremity. *Centruroides* stings are usually acutely painful, with a hypersensitive zone soon developing around the site. The injured area may be sensitive to touch, pressure, heat, and cold. Salivation, diaphoresis, perioral paresthesias, dysphagia, gastric distention, hyperactivity, diplopia, nystagmus, visual loss, incontinence, penile erection, exaggerated reflexes, abdominal pain, opisthotonos, hypertension (more common), hypotension (less common), pulmonary edema, coma, and muscle paralysis (including respiratory paralysis) can ensue, especially in children. Most nonlethal symptoms last less than four hours.

Treatment includes evaluation and application of cold to the sting site. Clean the site and apply a sterile, or at least clean, dressing. For severe pain, splint or immobilize the affected extremity. Oral, nonnarcotic analgesics may be useful. If serious symptoms develop (see above), immediate evacuation is indicated. If possible, bring the scorpion along on the evacuation, but avoid direct handling.

For those with the skill and equipment, benzodiazepine may be used for seizures and excitability. Methocarbamol may be administered IV for severe muscle spasms. Oral or parenteral antihypertensive medications (such as clonidine) may be required. If there are profound cholinergic effects, administer atropine. Give IV fluids carefully, if needed, since pulmonary edema may develop. Observe all healthy adults for at least four hours after a sting. Admit to the hospital all children and elderly patients stung by scorpions.

Administer IV antivenin only in cases of severe poisoning. It is available in most areas where dangerous scorpions exist. In the United States, it is only available in Arizona. Test for sensitivity to the serum only if the antivenin is to be used. Supportive care is considered by some authorities to be more important than the use of antivenin. Administer tetanus immunization.

D. Centipede Bites

Centipedes are found all over the United States. They rarely cause serious injury to humans. The giant desert centipede, which may attain a length of 15 cm (6 inches), can give a painful bite. Most bite reactions are local and no fatalities have been documented, but renal failure has been reported. Generally, centipedes hide in dark places. Check shoes, clothing, and bedding before use while traveling in centipede-infested areas.

Local reactions to centipede bites, in addition to intense pain, may include edema and erythema, lasting four to twelve hours. In severe bites, tenderness may persist or recur. To prevent secondary infection, cleanse the wound with soap and water. Apply cold and/or give oral analgesics for pain. In more serious reactions, where there is local lymphangitis, evidence of local necrosis at the bite site, or the rare systemic reaction, evacuate the patient. In case there is severe pain, infiltrate locally with lidocaine.

For centipede bites, observe patients with minor reactions for approximately four hours, or until the reaction improves. Admit patients with evidence of significant reaction to the hospital because of potential rhabdomyolysis and acute renal failure. Tetanus prophylaxis should be current.

Millipedes do not bite, but they may have secretions that irritate the skin. Treat by washing with soap and water (not alcohol) and applying a corticosteroid cream or lotion.

Chapter 22

TICK-TRANSMITTED DISEASES

I. GENERAL INFORMATION

Ticks transmit several serious illnesses to people. The most common infections are Lyme disease, Rocky Mountain spotted fever, relapsing fever, Colorado tick fever, and tick paralysis. In the Western Hemisphere, uncommon illnesses include Powassan encephalitis, babesiosis, tularemia, and ehrlichiosis.

II. PREVENTION

Several measures lessen the likelihood of acquiring a tick or a tick-borne illness. Clothing should be light-colored so that ticks can be more easily seen. Wear long-sleeved shirts and long pants. Tuck trousers inside a pair of high socks. Avoid contact with brush, if possible. Apply 0.5% permethrin tick repellent to clothing prior to exposure, with particular attention to the ends of shirt sleeves, pants, and collar area. A repellent containing DEET may be applied to the skin in the same areas and in other exposed locations, but overuse should be avoided, especially in children. A concentration of DEET no greater than 35% is recommended. Newer preparations containing synergists allow concentrations of less than 12% to be extremely effective. A controlled release formulation of DEET is available in 20% concentration that has been shown to significantly reduce absorption. Perform a full-body inspection for ticks daily. Wash clothing after exposure.

Ticks may not attach themselves for several hours after initial skin contact and until then they can be easily removed. Showering or bathing may remove unattached ticks. Once they have attached themselves, removal is substantially more difficult. Because transmission of infection is frequently delayed following tick attachment, remove attached ticks immediately when discovered.

No simple, effective method is known to cause the tick to detach itself. A good method of tick removal is to gently grasp the animal with tweezers as close as possible to the point of attachment, and remove by applying gentle, direct traction. A small piece of skin may come off pain-lessly with the tick, which usually means that tick removal is complete. It is not always possible to remove the mouthparts with the rest of the tick. If mouthparts remain, attempt to remove them with a needle or knife-point to avoid subsequent skin infection or inflammation. Avoid crushing the tick and contaminating either patient or helper with crushed tick material. Clean the wound with soap and water, and apply a bandage. Disinfect tweezers after use.

III. GUIDELINES FOR ASSESSMENT AND TREATMENT

A. Lyme Disease

Lyme disease is a recognized, widespread, tick-borne inflammatory illness caused by the *Borrelia burgdorferi* spirochete. In the United States, areas of high risk are the Northeast, the upper Midwest, California, southern Oregon, and western Nevada. Most bites occur between May 1 and November 30. The first abnormality is often an expanding circular red rash (erythema chronicum migrans), which occurs around the site where the tick was attached. Flu-like symptoms often develop shortly after the rash appears.

Disseminated infection, manifested by multiple annular secondary rashes, neurologic abnormalities (meningitis, Bell's palsy, peripheral neu-ropathy), arthralgias, and heart involvement (most commonly AV block) may occur beginning several weeks after the tick bite.

Months after an untreated infection, arthritis may develop, usually affecting the knees and shoulders. Persistent and varied neurologic abnor-malities may occur and persist for years.

Early treatment shortens the duration of erythema migrans and diminishes the likelihood of secondary and tertiary sequelae. Effective drugs at different stages of the disease are doxycycline, amoxicillin, ceftri-axone, and penicillin G. A new prophylactic immunization against Lyme disease is available for use in high-risk areas of the United States for per-sons fifteen to seventy years of age.

B. Rocky Mountain Spotted Fever

In many areas of the United States (especially Montana, Oklahoma, Missouri, and the Carolinas), ticks transmit rickettsia causing Rocky Mountain spotted fever, an illness characterized initially by fever, headache, sensitivity to bright light, and muscle aches. On the third to fourth day of fever, a pink rash usually appears. If not treated promptly with antibiotics (tetracycline), the disease may be lethal.

C. Relapsing Fever

Relapsing fever is an acute febrile illness caused by Borrelia spirochetes. *Ornithodoros* ticks that transmit relapsing fever do not usually attach to hosts but live in the host's nest or burrow and behave more like bedbugs. Wild rodents are the intermediate hosts. Clinically, initial symptoms are those of an acute flu-like illness, but bouts continue at weekly intervals. The diagnosis is established by identification of the organism in blood smears. Tetracycline and erythromycin are effective antibiotics. Prophylactically, one should avoid rodent-infested cabins.

D. Colorado Tick Fever

This disease is an acute benign viral infection that occurs throughout the Rocky Mountain area during spring and summer. It is characterized by fever, muscle aches, and headache. The white blood cell count is usually low. The fever is often biphasic, and lasts about one week. The diagnosis is confirmed by serologic testing. There is no specific therapy.

E. Tick Paralysis

Tick paralysis begins with leg weakness. An ascending flaccid paralysis follows, which worsens as long as the tick is attached to the patient (usually a child). Speech dysfunction and difficulty swallowing are late signs, and death from aspiration or respiratory paralysis may occur. Removal of the tick results in a progressive return to normal neurologic function. Both diagnostically and therapeutically, early meticulous examination for imbedded ticks is mandatory, especially near the hairline on the neck.

F. Babesiosis

Most infections are asymptomatic. Clinically evident disease presents with fever, chills, sweating, myalgias, fatigue, hepatosplenomegaly, and hemolytic anemia. Symptoms occur after an incubation period of one to four weeks and last several weeks. Disease due to *Babesia divergens* tends to be severe and is frequently fatal in immunosuppressed, splenectomized, or elderly patients. Clinical recovery usually occurs when infection is due to *B. microti*. The Medical Letter recommends antibiotic therapy with clindamycin and quinine, as well as other combinations of drugs in severely ill patients.

IV. CONTROVERSIES

Should prophylactic therapy be initiated following a tick bite in high-risk Lyme disease areas? Prophylactic therapy following a tick bite incurred in high risk areas is not recommended. The ticks (*Ixodes scapularis [dammini]*, *I. ricinus, I. pacificus*) carrying the germs that cause Lyme disease do not transmit the infection if attached for less than forty-eight hours.

Chapter 23

SUBSTANCE ABUSE IN WILDERNESS SETTINGS

I. GENERAL INFORMATION

Although data are sparse, it has been suggested that one of the single greatest contributing factors to trauma in wilderness areas is the nonprescribed and nonmedically indicated use of mood- and mind-altering chemicals. Substance abuse or misuse in wilderness settings appears to be responsible for significant morbidity and mortality from acute or chronic intoxication, accidental overdoses, and withdrawal.

II. GUIDELINES FOR ASSESSMENT AND TREATMENT

In any individual with an illness or injury in the wilderness, mind- or mood-altering drugs may complicate assessment and treatment. Consideration must be given to whether the patient's senses are so altered as to be unaware of his or her true physical state, including the presence of pain or imminent danger. If substance abuse is suspected, take extra time to assess the patient and give additional consideration to stabilization and care.

Working with people who are under the influence of drugs (including ethanol) is often difficult because such individuals may have radical alterations in personality, rapid mood swings, and irrational behavior patterns. A calm, unhurried, yet authoritative approach, especially with the use of a friend of the patient, can be effective in gaining the patient's confidence (or at least the patient's ear) and having him/her acquiesce to treatment.

In addition to the above, advanced providers may have two additional modalities: antidotes and sedation. Naloxone (0.4 to 4.0 mg IV, SQ), if available, will reverse the effects of narcotics and narcotic analogues. Sedation with antipsychotics (haloperidol) or benzodiazepines (diazepam, lorazepam) can be used if patients are in danger of harming themselves or others. Exercise extreme care to avoid depressing the respiratory drive in such individuals.

Chapter 24

ANXIETY AND STRESS REACTIONS IN THE WILDERNESS

I. GENERAL INFORMATION

Physical injury or accident in the wilderness, especially in severe cases, may be accompanied by significant psychological distress in the victim, in other party members, and even in rescuers. Panic and anxiety reactions are common in response to stressful situations. Other emotions may also occur, such as grief and depression. Victims or witnesses of traumatic injury may become so anxious that their safety (and that of other party members) is greatly compromised.

A critical incident is any situation faced by a trip participant that generates unusually strong emotional impact. These include: 1) the serious injury or death of a fellow participant; 2) the serious injury or death of a bystander; 3) multiple deaths or serious injuries; 4) serious injury or death of a child or infant; 5) any situation that attracts an unusual amount of attention from the media; 6) loss of life; and 7) any situation that is charged with emotion and causes an emotional response that is beyond the normal coping mechanisms of trip members.

An immediate stress reaction is the response of a normal person to an abnormal situation; it is not a sign of any psychological weakness or chronic psychiatric problems. The immediate stress reaction may include physical, emotional, cognitive, and behavioral components.

II. GUIDELINES FOR IMMEDIATE CARE IN THE FIELD

Medical care for physical injuries and securing the safety of all party members should take first priority in response to a wilderness accident. But just as one treats for shock while performing first aid or rescue operations, the psychological treatment of anxiety and stress reactions can begin almost immediately. Some basic procedures to consider in anxiety management include the following:

1) *Engage the patient in calm, rational discussion* while maintaining a focus on things that are improving (or making progress) during the first aid or rescue.
2) *Listen! Identify the specific concerns* about which the patient is anxious, and gently show that you, too, are concerned.
3) Provide realistic/optimistic feedback. When panic strikes, people often fear the worst and need to be brought back to objective thinking in the here-and-now.
4) *Use behavioral relaxation procedures,* especially if the patient is hyperventilating, to reduce somatic nervous system arousal; e.g., guide him or her through slow, deep breathing.
5) *Use guided imagery procedures,* such as word-pictures of pleasant events or places, to help reduce the pain.
6) *Involve the patient to the degree desired,* and to the degree possible, in actively participating in any decisions that must be made.
7) *Talk the patient through any technical skills* that he or she must participate in, with step-by-step advice.

III. MEDICATIONS

First-choice drugs for anxiety reduction are the benzodiazepines, such as diazepam, chlordiazepoxide, and alprazolam. While many drugs are effective for the symptomatic relief of anxiety (e.g., alcohol, barbiturates, and narcotic analgesics), the benzodiazepines are much safer. The primary side effect is mild sedation and, apart from potential interactions with other sedative drugs, there are very few contraindications. Therapeutic onset for anxiety relief takes from one to three hours (diazepam is the fastest acting) with typical oral dosages. Haldol given 5 mg to 10 mg (IM or PO) is also effective in treating this disorder.

IV. REFERRAL AND FOLLOW-UP

Victims of traumatic events, as well as their rescuers, are at increased risk of developing posttraumatic stress disorder (PTSD); therefore, they should be educated about major symptoms that signify the need for additional treatment. Primary symptoms of PTSD include 1) distressing dreams or reliving of the trauma; 2) persistent avoidance, psychogenic amnesia, or numbing in response to trauma-related stimuli; and 3) increased somatic nervous system arousal or hypervigilance. Any or all of these symptoms are part of the normal human reaction to trauma, but their persistence beyond a month is diagnostic of PTSD.

Clinical psychologists and psychiatrists who specialize in anxiety/stress disorders have developed some of the most effective treatments within recent years. Certain cognitive-behavioral therapies and particular drugs have proven effective, alone and in various combinations. The choice of specific psychotherapeutic or pharmacologic treatment will depend on the case and type of disorder.

V. OTHER CONSIDERATIONS

Emotional and behavioral disorders (or psychiatric illnesses, in medical nomenclature) are common in the general adult population with incidence rates in the general adult population of 10 percent for anxiety disorders, 6 percent for major depression, and at least 5 percent for personality disorders. Although mountain climbers and other wilderness adventurers may be robust and seem resistant to emotional distress, some expedition members might develop psychological problems. Most people undergo emotional changes in harsh environments, and personal conflicts often add stress to group dynamics. Thus, the success of a wilderness expedition depends in part on the "people skills" of the leader or other group member.

Chapter 25

WILDERNESS MEDICAL KITS

I. GENERAL INFORMATION

Preparations for wilderness activities include provisions for emergency care of individuals in the event of injuries or illnesses. Trip medical leaders must be able to assemble medical kits that are appropriate to support the proposed trip. This requires assessing several factors:

A. Purpose of the Trip

Selectivity is the key in choosing appropriate medical equipment. Groups intent only on providing self-treatment should consider the most common injuries they will sustain. Because a search and rescue (SAR) team must be equipped to handle the medical emergencies that they expect to encounter, they can justify carrying specialized medical gear. On recreational trips, however, the medical kit displaces other equipment that might be needed. Hikers, white water enthusiasts, and climbers all need different medical kits to meet their specialized needs.

B. Level of Medical Training

It is inappropriate to include medications and equipment that no trip member has the requisite knowledge or experience to use safely. Trip members responsible for medical care of the group should have direct input into the contents of the medical kit. Levels of training and experience can differ widely among groups of physicians, nurses, and EMS personnel. A degree or license may not guarantee knowledge in any specific area. Pretrip training to supplement the knowledge base of the providers may be advisable.

C. Destination

The terrain, altitude, weather, propensity for endemic diseases, and other inherent dangers must be considered. Groups heading into remote areas where local inhabitants may request medical help must consider this potential demand on their supplies and must consider whether they intend to respond.

D. Length of Trip

The total time that the party must be supported from the kit affects its contents. Some problems are likely to occur only during particular times. For example, the treatment of friction blisters is most important during the first few days of a hike. At times on a long trip, outside medical supplies can be obtained to restock the kit.

E. Time for Evacuation or Medical Rescue

Some trips progressively distance themselves from medical care. On other trips, time required to obtain help may be deceptive. A river raft trip into a canyon, for instance, may last only hours, but evacuation in the event of an accident may require many days of dangerous and laborious effort.

F. Size of the Party

Although an increase in the number of participants influences the quantity of some medications and bandaging materials, the increase is not linear. Frequently, only minimal additions are needed to serve a larger group adequately. Equipping each member with a personal kit containing bandages, blister supplies, and personal medications can reduce the size of the main medical kit for a large party.

G. Bulk, Weight, and Cost

Even if cost is not a consideration, the weight and bulk of a kit are potential limiting factors. Because bandaging and splints are bulky and possibly awkward to carry, the use of improvised materials, such as clothing for bandaging and local fabrication of splints, may be incorporated into plans for the medical kit. Using multifunctional components may also reduce medical equipment. If one piece of equipment or a drug can be used for many different purposes, weight can be significantly reduced. Knowledgeable medical team members are needed to optimize this tactic.

Some organizations and search and rescue teams use a modular approach to medical kits. Separate kits, with increasing sophistication and for various purposes, are available for individuals and situations requiring more advanced equipment. While the basic kit is designed for use by lay personnel, only specially trained individuals can use the more advanced kits, and they carry them into the field only when required.

II. CONTAINERS

Containers for the medical kit must be chosen for maximal accessibility and protection of contents. Damage is to be expected and may render materials useless. In situations where there is danger of the loss of equipment, such as on white-water trips, the medical kit components should be divided into several kits so that all equipment is not lost if an accident occurs. Individuals with life-sustaining medications should take an extra quantity to be carried separately.

The medical kit must be easily identified and accessible when needed. This entails making it visible, e.g., bright red and/or marked with reflective material, and placing it where it can be reached easily. Kits that unroll or open to display their contents make selection of items very convenient. For small kits, this is not usually necessary. For large kits, kits that will be used frequently, and kits that may be accessed by multiple members of the group, accessibility and easy identification of contents are very important.

III. GUIDELINES FOR EQUIPMENT

Equipment for a wilderness medical kit should be selected in light of its function:

A. Life Support

Airways, supplemental oxygen, manually powered suction devices, and similar equipment are generally only carried by experienced rescue personnel on prolonged remote expeditions.

B. Vital Signs

A watch with a second hand to time pulse or respiration is an important piece of equipment. A blood pressure cuff and stethoscope are useful in some situations, but are of no value to untrained personnel.

C. Soft Tissue Injuries

An irrigation syringe will provide adequate wound cleaning capability. Wound closure materials range from butterfly bandages and wound closure strips to suture equipment with surgical instruments or surgical staples. Cleansing materials, local anesthetics, and bandaging materials are also in this category. Material for blister treatment is probably the most commonly used item in this group.

D. Orthopedic Injuries

Prefabricated splints are now manufactured in lightweight designs, including collapsible femoral traction splints, but these may be improvised in the field. Cervical collars may likewise be improvised. Backboards or litters are not usually needed, except by rescue groups. Fiberglass casting material makes an excellent lightweight splinting material.

E. Medication Administration

Special equipment in addition to the medications is necessary only if injectable drugs or intravenous fluids are carried. Injectable medications are susceptible not only to damage from bottle breakage, but also from light, heat, and cold.

IV. MEDICATIONS

The decision to carry any particular medication must take into account the medical knowledge required to use the medication properly, as well as the cost, bulk, and weight of the kit, the potential problems that might be encountered, medication allergy history of trip participants, and knowledge of local laws and regulations that might restrict possession of certain medications.

A list of potential candidates for inclusion in this list can be obtained by referring to suggestions made in these position papers, various books on wilderness-related medical care, the physician's personal medical/surgical knowledge, and standard texts and publications concerning treatment of trauma and infectious diseases. The Wilderness Medicine Letter and *The Journal of Wilderness & Environmental Medicine,* publications of the Wilderness Medical Society, periodically publish articles with suggestions for customized medical kits for various remote area, climatic, and endeavor-specific activities.

Chapter 26

IMMUNIZATIONS

GENERAL INFORMATION

Appropriate immunizations are vital for those entering wilderness and foreign areas. Current recommendations for U.S. travelers are issued by the Centers for Disease Control and Prevention (CDC), published annually in *Health Information for International Travel*. The publication contains vaccination and certification requirements for malaria and yellow fever on a country-by-country basis. It also includes the U.S. Public Health Service recommendations for difficult immunization questions, such as immunization of infants and pregnant or lactating women, and specific recommendations for vaccination and prophylaxis for a wide variety of disorders. It also contains a discussion of specific potential health hazards worldwide, grouped by geographic region. The information in this book is updated in the biweekly *Summary of Health Information for International Travel*. Both the book and updates can be obtained from the Superintendent of Documents, U.S. Government Printing Office, Washington, DC 20402. A weekly report of infectious diseases in the United States and important overseas medical developments is contained in the CDC publication *Morbidity and Mortality Weekly Report*. Subscriptions can be obtained from the CDC, Atlanta, GA 30333, or from the Massachusetts Medical Society, C.S.P.O. Box 9120, Waltham, MA 02254-9120, which reprints these reports as part of an inexpensive subscription service.

The Centers for Disease Control and Prevention has a hotline that provides twenty-four-hour information on current disease status: (404) 639-1610. A fax service is also available through this number that will return information concerning malaria prophylaxis and other disease risk factors. Access the CDC via the Internet at www.cdc.gov/travel.

The Department of State has a twenty-four-hour hotline that provides general country information, with a travel risk assessment, at (202) 647-5225. Contact the Department of State via the Internet at www.travel.state.gov/travel_warnings.

An alternative source of information is *Vaccination Certificate Requirements and Health Advice for International Travelers*, published yearly by the World Health Organization, Geneva, Switzerland. It is available through the WHO Publication Center U.S.A., 49 Sheridan Avenue, Albany, NY 12210. Contact the WHO via the Internet at www.who.int.

The local county or state board of health will frequently have information from the above sources available for consultation and/or will have a referral service to local travel medicine specialists.

Current immunization advice, disease risk charts, and other information concerning the availability of medical care within foreign countries can be obtained from IAMAT (International Association for Medical Assistance to Travelers), 417 Center St., Lewistown, NY 14092, (716) 754–4883. IAMAT provides this information to travelers and physicians free of charge, operating only with donations. Contact IAMAT via the Internet at www.sentex.net/~iamat.

The Scope of Wilderness Medicine

Our interests include the following areas:

- Physiologic interactions of environmental forces on human performance and health
- Environmental health disorders
    Heat illness
    Hypothermia, hyperthermia
    Frostbite
    Altitude illness
    Barotrauma submersion
- Health risks in specific environments
    Mountains
    Deserts
    Jungles
    Marine
    Aerospace
    Subterranean (caves)
- Health risks from plants and animals
    Toxinology
    Animal attacks
- Traditional medicine in remote environments
    Wilderness trauma
    Medical limitations to wilderness travel
- Travel medicine
- Medical services in wilderness settings
    Search and rescue
    Organization of wilderness medical services
    Expedition medicine
- Infectious diseases from the wilderness and foreign travel
- Liability in wilderness medicine
- Education in wilderness medicine
- Global health issues from environmental depredation

Share Our Members' Sense of Adventure

   Our physician and professional members are committed to expanding their knowledge of the prevention, diagnosis, and treatment of wilderness diseases and injuries.

   Society members include experts in high-altitude physiology and medical problems from exposure to heat and cold. Others work with astronauts and aquanauts or treat the victims of animal attacks, poisonous bites, and stings. Many WMS members play an integral role in wilderness medical issues within government, civic, and medical organizations.

Mission Statement

The purpose of the Wilderness Medical Society is to encourage, foster, support, or conduct activities or programs concerned with life sciences that can improve the scientific knowledge of the membership and the general public in matters related to wilderness environments and human activities in these environments.

The mission of the Wilderness Medical Society is to establish an organization composed of qualified physicians, allied health specialists and other qualified individuals that will concern itself with matters related to wilderness medicine and the benefits, health, safety, and medical care of the individual in the wilderness.

Dear Wilderness Medicine Enthusiast,

This is your special invitation to join the Wilderness Medical Society, the largest organization in the world devoted to wilderness medical issues. The Society is traditional in its commitment to medical knowledge, education, and research. Yet, it is unique in its focus on wilderness environments and the challenges they present.

As a Society member, you will join physicians and other professionals who share medical, conservation, and recreational interest in wilderness activities. You will have a wealth of opportunities and materials for professional and personal growth such as clinical journals, publications, slide-lecture sets, and accredited scientific meetings. In addition, you will have ample opportunity to play a leadership role in the Society.

Regular membership in the Wilderness Medical Society is an outstanding value at only $100 per year, which includes your journal subscription. Other membership categories include the newsletter and the option to subscribe to the journal. Whether you are an accomplished wilderness traveler and an expert in wilderness medicine or you are just beginning to cultivate your interest in the field, the Wilderness Medical Society is for you.

We look forward to your favorable reply.

Cordially,

The Board of Directors
Wilderness Medical Society

Membership Application

Please complete the form below and mail it along with the dues for the appropriate membership category to: Wilderness Medical Society, 3595 East Fountain Boulevard, Suite A1, Colorado Springs, CO 80910. Phone: (719) 572-9255; Fax: (719) 572-1514.

NAME _____ DATE_____

ADDRESS _____

CITY_____

STATE _____ ZIP_____

TELEPHONE HOME _____

BUSINESS FAX _____

E-MAIL _____

My primary interest in the Wilderness Medical Society is: _____
_____

How did you find out about the Wilderness Medical Society?_____
_____

Medical specialty, if any _____

_____ Regular member $100/year, (includes journal subscription)

_____ Associate/Student member $33/year

_____ Associate/Student member with journal subscription $83/year

_____ Life member—$2,000/year

_____ Corporate member—$1,000/year

M/C OR VISA NO. _____

EXPIRATION DATE _____ SIGNATURE _____

WILDERNESS MEDICAL SOCIETY

3595 East Fountain Boulevard

Colorado Springs, CO 80910

Phone: (719) 572-9255

Fax: (719) 572-1514

E-mail: wms@wms.org

Visit the WMS Web site at www.wms.org for more information about conferences, membership, books, educational slide sets, and more!

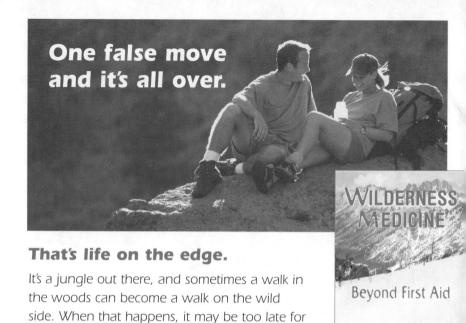

One false move and it's all over.

That's life on the edge.

It's a jungle out there, and sometimes a walk in the woods can become a walk on the wild side. When that happens, it may be too late for Band-Aid measures. What you really need is some basic knowledge of first aid and survival techniques.

The Globe Pequot Press can provide the basics (and a lot of specifics) if you think you could use a "crash course" in practical wilderness first-aid treatment.

You can provide the T.L.C.

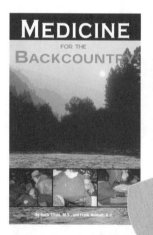

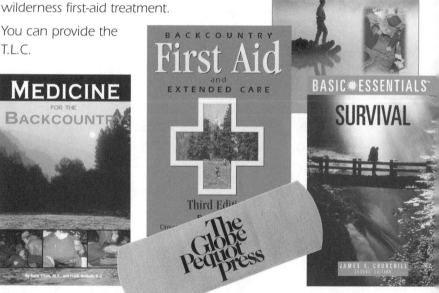

WILDERNESS MEDICINE

Beyond First Aid

The WILDERNESS FIRST RESPONDER

a text for the recognition, treatment and prevention of wilderness emergencies

BACKCOUNTRY
First Aid
and
EXTENDED CARE

Third Edition

The Globe Pequot Press

BASIC ✴ ESSENTIALS™
SURVIVAL

JAMES E. CHURCHILL